THE DOCTOR NEXT DOOR

"This book is a refreshing compilation of stories about the true meaning of why many physicians choose to become doctors. Dr. Holt epitomizes compassion and bedside manner and emphasizes the importance of refocusing medicine away from science and back to the art of caring and being a doctor."

—ANDREW JACONO, MD, FACS

"In an era of impressive, but impersonal technology, Dr. Holt reminds us what is at the core of true healing: the patient/physician relationship. With inquiry, insight, and a dash of aplomb; her stories refresh the reader's spirit, and give us hope that despite the augers, the human touch will remain the heart and soul of healing."

—CHEF MICHAEL FENSTER, MD; "The Food Shaman"

"It is true talent when a writer can take something as technical as medical science and make it engaging and inspirational for the reader. Dr. Holt brings that talent to life in *The Doctor Next Door* which she makes clear in her opening words that, 'real medicine isn't about science. It's about people and their stories . . .' And, she does that so well on every page whether she is sharing a vignette about a patient, their family, or even other medical staff. "

—DAVID MEZZAPELLE, Author of the bestselling *Contagious Optimism* book series

Openness

The Doctor Next Door

by Elaine Holt, M.D.

ISBN 978-1-63393-576-1

Published by

◀ köehlerbooks™

210 60th Street
Virginia Beach, VA 23451
800-435-4811
www.koehlerbooks.com

THE DOCTOR NEXT DOOR

ELAINE HOLT, M.D.

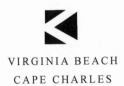

VIRGINIA BEACH
CAPE CHARLES

TABLE OF CONTENTS

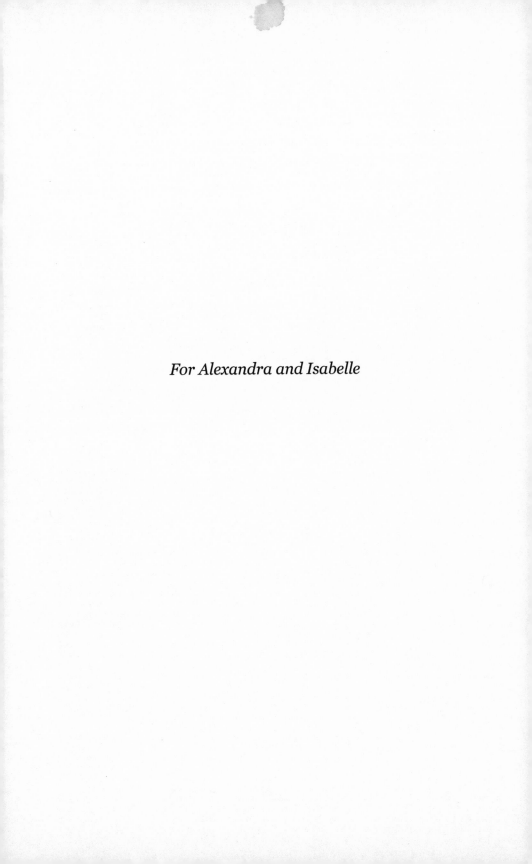

For Alexandra and Isabelle

NOTE TO THE READER

I hope that you will enjoy these patient encounters as much as I did, and I hope that you will learn from them the same way that I have tried to. I have changed all patient names and identifying characteristics to preserve confidentiality. All of the dialogue included in this book has been reconstructed by me through my memory of the events so it is unlikely to represent verbatim conversations.

I have, however, tried to stay true to the shared feelings and dynamics of the relationships revealed and have done my best to invite you into some memorable experiences. At times I have merged encounters that in fact may have occurred years apart and have taken some creative liberties in the interest of storytelling. Please know that, above all, I am grateful to the patients who have shared and who continue to share their lives with me and it is through them that I have grown wiser.

INTRODUCTION

Most doctors go into medicine with good intentions. They want to help people. I was no different. However, I had no idea that I'd end up getting as much from my patients as I'd be giving to them. You see, real medicine isn't about science. It's about people and their stories.

The Doctor Next Door is a collection of stories based on my decades of Internal Medicine practice. It celebrates the doctor-patient relationship, personal relationships, and the resilience of the human spirit. My hope is that these extraordinary stories of ordinary people will inspire you, as they've inspired me.

As a solo practitioner swimming against the tide of corporatized medicine, I believe in the intimacy of the doctor-patient bond and I've based my career on its enduring strength.

Now, you might be wondering who I am. My patients refer to me as a modern day throwback to the small-town doctor.

I was raised in a family who believed in keeping elderly relatives at home as their health, minds, and bodies declined. As a result, when it came time to assess what I wanted to be when I grew up, I had only to reflect on what I'd already become—a caregiver. I had been a "feeder" to an aging grandparent, preparing meals and spoon-feeding for as long as I can remember. Fortunately, I didn't have a naysaying guidance counselor or meddling parent telling me that my choice didn't make sense.

After completing my residency training in Internal Medicine in New York City, I embarked on my career as a private practice physician and have spent the last seventeen years as a custodian of patients and their stories.

A while back I found out that one of my patients, a priest, had just accepted a position at a new parish. Not knowing whether this was a promotion of sorts in his line of work, I said, "Father, congratulations on the new parish . . . It's quite a career accomplishment."

He replied, "Oh, I don't really think of it as a career. It's more like a calling, you understand."

Reflecting on my own choices, I answered, "I think I do."

Chapter One

THERE'S NOTHING YOU CAN'T RECOVER FROM . . .

I was sitting with a friend
In a drugstore parking lot
We were waiting for another
In this designated spot.

Each of us discouraged
About the station of our life
Him—concern about his future
Me—a relationship in strife.

When he, a wise and thoughtful soul
said "I have advice. I'll give you some.
Don't be afraid of what will be
There's nothing you can't recover from."

This thought was said with nonchalance
Long conceived by him as fact.
A concept not yet known to me
Insight into this I lacked.

Don't stay in stale relationships
'Cause you're afraid of what won't be
Know that after the initial hurt
A stronger you you'll see.

If your job is unfulfilling
And your outlook has grown bleak
"There's nothing you can't recover from."
A new job you should seek

I reflect back on that time
A lightbulb moment then was flashed
"There's nothing you can't recover from."
All future fears at once were dashed.

***

I was working in a group practice at the time in which each doctor functioned on his or her personal island. Each physician had his/her own receptionist or scheduler and a nurse representative. Of course, it would have been more cost-effective to share the staff and stagger schedules, but the group was about as cohesive as a pack of wild dogs. To prevent our inevitable in-fighting, we created multiple distinct offices in one. There were so many staffers, we wordlessly walked down hallways turning sideways when passing one another to avoid any accidental physical contact. But, ironically, in the interest of cost-containment, we rented a small office space with narrow corridors and a single bathroom. Go figure.

Believe it or not, we existed for years like this and were able to somewhat seamlessly service the local community and suppress our pathologies long enough to sign out clinical concerns at the end of the shift. This aseptic "sign-out" was as close as we came to speaking. I know how absurd this must sound, but doctors can be strong-willed characters addicted to having a say just for the sake of it. You don't make it through the rigors of medical school and residency by being the shy, retiring type.

So, distinct, colorful personalities of different generations, genders, and cultures tried to unite in too small an office space for the sake of treating the local community. Tensions ran high.

Being the newest physician to join the group, I often got last dibs on office space, exam rooms, and clinical staff. I was originally paired with a nurse who looked good on paper. Her name was Gwen, and she had all of the right credentials: diplomas from fine schools, license in order, fifteen years of experience—so not a novice, but not so old that she might be jaded. Unfortunately, it was a "love the one you're with" relationship between me and Gwen. She, as an employee, had no choice of doctor and I, as a newbie, had no choice of assistant, so we were paired.

Gwen made efforts to appear the model employee. She came to work early and left late. In fact, I remember one of the senior partners remarking on what a find Gwen was at several weekly office meetings. It was this senior partner, after all, who had hired Gwen, so the fact that she was seemingly working out was fodder for self-congratulations.

I had my doubts about Gwen. She'd be sullen and sulky one minute and bubbly and chatty the next. Some days she'd join the staff at the communal lunch table. Other days she preferred to stay in her cubicle working intently on her phone. Her resume was extensive, but I didn't see the consistency of experience reflected in her day-to-day performance. I was reluctant to say anything at our office meetings as the slightest digression from the agenda could prolong them in excess of their already painful sixty-minute slot in the schedule.

So, Gwen continued to come early, around 6:45 a.m. for an 8:00 a.m. start of the day. I was an early bird as well and would routinely arrive at work to find Gwen waiting to be let in. Only the doctors had keys to the office. That senior partner mentioned earlier preferred to do paperwork after official hours and would lock up shortly after Gwen left. So, that's how she got in at 6:45 a.m. and out at 6:45 p.m. Any rational person would now be wondering why a salaried employee was working a twelve-hour day instead of an eight-hour one.

Did I mention that in addition to being stubborn and willful, doctors can also be naive and gullible? We assume that if you've chosen healthcare as your profession, you are selflessly dedicated and your hard work and tenacity are born out of a deep devotion to changing lives. Ha!

It wasn't until I mounted evidence that I brought my concerns to the group. Gwen was in charge of making telephone calls to my patients and informing them of results. On several different occasions, patients would page me after hours looking for results that I was certain I'd asked Gwen to report several business days ago. *What the hell was she doing during a twelve hour day if not addressing my phone calls?* I asked myself. She would write a weight down in the chart as part of taking vital signs and I'd go in the exam room, chart in hand, and say cheerfully: "Congratulations! You've lost twelve pounds." The patient would look confused and say, "Nobody weighed me."

That bitch, I mused to myself as I gestured grandly to the scale suggesting that we go ahead and weigh now.

Another curiosity about Gwen was her bathroom regimen. She seemed to have a "sensitive stomach," as your grandmother might have put it. Someone less discreet might have called it an unpredictable and relentless case of the runs followed ceremoniously by retching and vomiting. Did I mention already that there was only one bathroom in our suite? Adjacent offices were constantly being called upon by the receptionists as they asked to use their facilities. I couldn't blame them. I, myself, was developing "teacher's bladder," a condition of a chronically distended bladder from holding urine for an unreasonable length of time. Anything was better than confronting our bowl, uniquely splattered with pink flecks of undigested food or speckled with watery, brown droplets extending unnaturally beyond the toilet's rim.

And so were things at the suburban doctor's office until one day, the receptionist fielded a call from a local pharmacist. The pharmacist asked to speak to me directly and was not interested in talking to a doctor's representative.

"Hello," I answered warily. Pharmacists are, as a general rule, not overly chatty so I feared that he'd discovered a medication error or wanted to report some mistake in drug dispensing.

"Hi, Dr. Holt?" he inquired.

"Yes," I confirmed.

"This is Jim from such and such pharmacy. I'm calling to verify a recent prescription called in under your name and license number."

"Sure. Go ahead," I said and instinctively closed my office door with my free hand.

"Were you aware of a prescription for Percocet, strength 5/325, called into this pharmacy on Monday of last week for Gwen X in the quantity of one hundred tablets?"

I stammered a bit and said, "No."

"Then I take it you're not aware of the prescription for Percocet, strength 7.5/325, called into pharmacy "y" in the amount of sixty tablets on x date?"

"No."

"How about a prescription for Percocet called in on the same date into pharmacy 'z'? That amount was strength 10/325 for forty-five tablets all for Gwen X."

"Nope! Who was the call-in representative?" I asked, trying to piece this together.

"It varied. Sometimes it was Ann. Sometimes it was Jennifer," he answered. These were all other nurses or healthcare representatives in the office authorized to phone in prescriptions. I thought to myself, *What a bunch of fools we are!* All this time we had thought Gwen, nurse extraordinaire, was coming in early and leaving late to get a leg up on her work when really, her extended hours allowed her to access the phones to call in her fraudulent prescriptions without being overheard.

Like a bee in a jar, I darted from one office to the next trying to find my physician partners, one of whom I hadn't spoken to in a calendar year except for those aforementioned patient sign-outs. This kind of information justified a lifting of our word ration and a swift exchange of information. It was decided that Gwen would be terminated immediately and we would try to facilitate her getting help.

Gwen being dismissed rid me of a manipulative and inefficient assistant, but it also left me high and dry with no replacement. It was going to be hard to keep up a busy office schedule, run two exam rooms simultaneously and address patient calls in a timely manner without an assistant.

As I said, it was every doctor for his or herself at this office, and I knew that it would be a matter of days before I started to feel rushed and behind schedule without additional manpower. Hiring a new employee seemed like a job for a human resources team versed in local newspaper ads and Internet postings, but, in a physician-owned practice, hiring a new employee was the doctor's responsibility. There's endless paperwork built into the very fabric of medicine as it is, and I couldn't conceive of inviting more tedium into my day by sifting through responses from a widely distributed job advertisement. I shuddered at the thought of being buried alive by reams of CVs as they spilled out of the fax paper tray onto the floor, engulfing the receptionist area with eight-inch by ten-inch accounts of people's accomplishments.

It would be like Strega Nona and the spaghetti swallowing the town except I would have no magic pasta pot to halt the process. So, the decision was made— no advertisement.

Just as I was fatiguing on asking little old ladies if they had a grandkid in nursing or asking middle aged folks if that son or daughter of theirs had ever secured a job after college graduation, my luck began to turn: Joe came in for an earache.

I had seen Joe only once before for a strep throat swab and really didn't know him well. He was young and handsome and seemed quite unassuming. He stood six feet, two inches tall, but never struck me as that big until that day. Perhaps that was because I usually greeted people once they were already seated, but now that I was without Gwen, I was rooming my own patients directing them from the lobby into the exam rooms. (This exercise confirmed for me why I never worked as a hostess in the food service industry.) So, this was the first time I'd seen Joe stand up. He towered over me as he gestured for me to enter the exam room first and I "mock ducked" as I went under his arm which was holding the door ajar.

"So what can we do for you, sir?" I asked, holding a thermometer under his tongue.

"Just hold that thought. These oral, electronic ones take a while, but they're better than the alternative."

He smiled without parting his lips, as it would dislodge the temperature probe.

"Good. No fever. So let's try again. What brings you?" I asked.

"My ear. The right one. I've been doing a lot of flying and it hurt quite a bit on takeoff and landing this last time," he answered.

"Flying where? Anywhere good?" I said assembling the otoscope and looking in the good ear. You always look in the "good ear" first so you have a baseline for comparison.

"Some travel for work. I just got back from Nebraska."

"Wow, this ear looks red. No membrane rupture though." I

took my seat on the rolling stool, checked the chart for antibiotic allergies, and began writing his prescription.

"What's in Nebraska?" I asked, not averting my eyes from my prescription pad.

"Besides the Central Lowlands and the Great Plains?" he said, clearly proud of his home state.

"Yes, besides those notable landforms."

"Well, I'm from there originally. I also accompanied a friend of mine back for a visit."

"A friend?" I asked inquisitively with one eyebrow raised.

"Just a friend," he assured me with a bashful blush. "We're from the same town in Nebraska and she relocated here a year ago with a buddy of mine. They were going to get married, but things didn't work out."

"Oh, I'm sorry to hear that. It's hard to move to a new place and have your relationship status change at the same time."

"I know. She and I have been friends since grammar school. It would have been cool if they stayed together. I'm friends with both of them, you know. So, it's a balancing act until the dust settles."

"Well, she's lucky to have you to lean on."

"It was a fun trip. At first she was going to move right back to Nebraska once they called off the engagement, but then she decided to stick around here while she applied to medical school. I'm just trying to be supportive," he said.

I don't think I heard anything past "medical school," and in my head I saw myself as a shark circling the bloody waters— hopefully I didn't look quite as hungry on the outside.

"Did you just say that your friend will be applying to medical school?"

"Yes. She wants to stay around here for her gap year and see what happens after that. It's easier than going back home and moving again."

"Really? "I'm looking for an assistant. Do you think that's something she'd be interest in?"

"Gosh. I'm sure she would love to interview with you. She worked in her dad's OB/GYN office in Nebraska, so she's even had some medical office experience," he answered excitedly.

Who says "gosh" anymore besides Opie on The Andy Griffith *show?* I asked myself. There was a charming innocence about this young man and I wanted to be able to help him help his friend.

"Joe, this sounds like it could be a love connection. Let's see what we can do to get her over here. What's her name?"

"Maggie. Margaret actually, but she goes by Maggie. Wow, this is great news," he remarked, proud that he'd made this contact for his friend in need. I handed him my business card along with his prescription and asked him to have Maggie forward her résumé. I told him that I was ready to interview and make decisions about the hire right away so she shouldn't delay in reaching out to me. What I declined to mention was that Maggie was my only interviewee and that I was about to resort to taking pennies out of the fountain in the center of town and tossing them at passersby to draft other candidates. Internally preoccupied, I didn't hear him the first time he tried to thank me. Clearing his throat, he extended his hand for a firm shake.

"Dr. Holt, thank you sooo much. Maggie's a great girl. You're going to love her. And I want to thank you for giving her an opportunity to interview here."

"My pleasure, Joe. Truly it is. Have her reach out to me and we'll set up a time to meet soon. In the meantime, let me know if that antibiotic doesn't clear up your ear. You're not flying again soon, right?" I asked.

"No. I'm grounded for a while. I'll give Maggie a ring when I leave here. Thanks again."

"No problem," I said and hoped that he'd gauged his friend's potential interest accurately. It didn't take long to hear from

Maggie. Her résumé was on the fax when I arrived the next morning. I was able to reach her by phone at lunchtime and set up an interview later that week.

I had arranged for her to come in at lunchtime so that the morning appointments would have been over and my partners would either be rounding at the hospital or holed up in their respective offices doing paperwork. My mission was accomplished because I was the only one in the back office when Maggie arrived. I'd let my favorite receptionist in on the interview, so she shuttled her back without anyone asking any questions. You wouldn't think that interviewing a new staffer would need to be a covert mission, but frankly, I didn't want any unsolicited commentary from my colleagues. I stood and reached over my desk to shake her hand and was instantly struck by our difference in height. She stood at least six inches taller than I and I thought to myself, *what an odd pairing we'd make at first glance.*

She was statuesque with beautiful, wavy brown hair streaked naturally with sunny highlights. Sunny was the right way to describe Maggie; her blue eyes opened wide with excitement and her face was animated even as she introduced herself. In that instant, I realized something important—a fact I would come back to over and over again in my own life. People like being around happy people.

Gwen, albeit drug-addicted and clearly troubled, had also been negative and depressing to be around. If she wasn't sick, she was tired. If she wasn't tired, she was unhappy. That kind of kvetching gets old. And here, before me like a stroke of good luck, born out of some idle patient chitchat was the adorable, upbeat potential answer to my most pressing professional woe.

Maggie dressed for the interview and I imagined conversations that she might have had earlier with her mother as she weighed in on the right "first impression" outfit. Maggie had settled on a two-piece, pencil-skirt ensemble. Her long torso did well with a peplum top that flared at the waist, giving the illusion of an hourglass figure and her pencil skirt was a charming throwback to something the ladies might have worn in the secretarial pools of the nineteen-fifties.

"So, Maggie, what brings you out this way?"

"Well, I'm from Nebraska originally," she answered flashing a straight smile—the product of caring parents and orthodontia. "But I like it here. I actually went to college out here," she said. This prompted me to scan her résumé for the college listing.

"And you're going to be taking a year off to apply to medical school?" I asked.

"Yes. I have all of my prerequisites done, and I've taken the MCAT. I'm just looking for a job out here while I apply, and a job in the medical field would be ideal,." She sat erect, at the edge of the seat, with her hands in her lap draped gracefully over a leather billfold that undoubtedly contained extra resumes, references, and other job interview paraphernalia. She struck me as catholic school educated, and I envisioned the nuns tapping her between the shoulder blades as a tactile reminder to sit up straight or throat-clearing while proctoring exams, urging Maggie to sit with both feet flat on the floor. Her imagined parochial schooling aside, Maggie seemed bright and eager and, maybe more important— available. She had something I wanted, and I had something she wanted: a perfect match. I asked perfunctory questions about her volunteer experience and learned more about her work duties in her dad's OB/GYN practice. It turned out that she'd worked on the ambulance corps in Nebraska and could take vital signs and give shots. Phlebotomy (blood drawing), a practiced skill, was the only duty of the job that we would iron out along the way. As it was, I had been doing my own phlebotomy since Gwen's untimely departure, so Maggie's novice status hardly seemed like a deal breaker.

As we were wrapping up the interview and I asked, "So

Maggie, how do you know Joe?"

With a smile, she said, "Joe? We went to grammar school together. We were in the same fifth grade class and we've been dear friends ever since."

"Did you go to high school together, too?"

"Yes, middle school and high school, but we went to different colleges. We saw each other on breaks and have kept up our friendship throughout the years."

"A patient told me once that friends come in three varieties: friends for a reason, friends for a season, and friends for a lifetime," I supplied.

"I've never heard that before, but I guess it's true,.."

"I'd like to think that some childhood friends can be friends for a lifetime. In any case, Joe spoke very highly of you and I'm glad that he was able to send you in my direction."

"Oh, me too. It was a pleasure meeting you."

"Likewise," I answered, rising out of my chair to see her to the door. "I just want to do my due diligence by checking your references." I no sooner asked then she was flipping open her leather billfold to produce a typed sheet of paper containing three references, two work and one personal. Her preparedness thrilled me and I knew that, barring anything untoward on the reference check, we would be working together.

True to form, she must have sent a thank you note later that afternoon from a local post office and I received it in the next day's mail. Her references were glowing and the deal was sealed. I wasted no time and reached her on her cell phone the next day to offer her the position.

"Maggie? It's Elaine Holt. How are you?" I asked.

"Oh fine, Dr. Holt. How are you? It's nice to hear from you," she answered and you could hear her anticipation.

"Maggie, your references are glowing, so you can pay them off now," I said. She laughed heartily and assured me that she'd do that as soon as we got off the phone.

"I was delighted to meet you, and I think that we'd work well together. I hope that an opportunity in this office would be a good learning experience for you as well," I said, subtly pitching the position.

"Oh, I know that it would be, and the folks I met seemed really nice," she assured. Little did she know that only a quarter of the staff had been present on her interview day, but she'd learn about the interoffice dynamics soon enough. We went over some of the logistics: the hours, the pay, and a loose job description.

"Sounds great!" she said without any objections or negotiations. To think that this lovely young lady was close friends with the "oh gosh" guy could make even a reluctant educator want to go back and teach in their elementary school in Nebraska.

"Great. I think we'll make a fine team. Welcome aboard. Now, when do you think you could start?" I asked.

"Well, as soon as I give notice at the daycare center I work at now. Maybe two or three weeks?" she asked tentatively.

"Ok, very good. So it's a deal, and keep me posted on your start date. Their loss is my gain," I answered.

"Thanks so much Dr. Holt. I really appreciate the opportunity, and I will definitely keep you posted. I'll be in touch soon."

"Looking forward to it."

She started two weeks later and, as expected, the transition was seamless. The staff loved her. Patients loved her. I loved her. Although there was a fifteen-year age difference, we interacted like peers. I, my favorite receptionist, and Maggie made up an island of endless twittering and banter. No topic of conversation was left untouched, from American Idol top picks to religion in schools. We flitted around the office in a finely coordinated relay to move through a packed patient schedule. It worked and it was fun. My greatest revenge for being burdened by Gwen's employment and then again burdened by Gwen's departure was my happiness with Maggie.

I knew that there was some divine doctor-patient karma to thank for it. If Joe hadn't had an earache when he did and if he hadn't come in for the appointment and if I hadn't asked him about his personal life, I would have never found Maggie. Thank you, doctor-patient karma! It would benefit me many times over in my career going forward.

I so enjoyed Maggie and my favorite receptionist's company that we started eating lunch together. Sometimes, it was just the three of us and at other times, the rest of the staff would join. The non-physician office staff was not afflicted with the same interpersonal conflicts that burdened the doctors, so the white flags could come out for an hour in the middle of the day. Each nurse-receptionist duo could abandon their post and their physician allegiance to sit at the rectangular lunch table together.

It was at this table that some wild if not thought-provoking exchanges took place. I remember a conversation about childbirth. One of the grandmothers-to-be of the bunch was reminiscing about her three "natural" childbirth experiences and how she hoped that large babies weren't inherited because her last had been an even ten pounds and she worried about her pregnant daughter.. She took the opportunity to pass around the twelve-week prenatal ultrasound picture.

"Oh, I wish I had one of these. I didn't have ultrasounds when I was carrying Karina. I just had a headache," said Jane, our phlebotomist. I'm sure I furrowed my brow in an obvious plea for clarity. Maggie looked to me just as I was poorly concealing my confusion and nearly spit string cheese out all over the table.

"Jane, what do you mean, you had a headache instead of an ultrasound? What are you saying?" I asked. At this point, my receptionist was breaking into her contagious giggles and the whole group of ladies had stopped eating and watched Jane expectantly.

"There was no time for an ultrasound. I went into the hospital with a headache and I came out with a baby," she answered matter-of-factly.

A series of loud "what's?" "Are you kidding's?" "What the hell are you talking about's?" were thrown out. Perhaps our exuberance got the best of us because one of the physician partners stuck her head out of the office admonishingly and shut her door so she could address her paperwork in greater serenity. Lowering her voice to a stage whisper, one of the other nurses asked, "Is this like an episode of Jerry Springer where the woman didn't know she was pregnant and delivered a baby in a toilet?! Please tell me that's not what this is?"

"I was young," Jane defended. This was all that was needed to bring professionalism to a halt. There was uncontrolled laughter, mouth covering disbelief, and heads hung in exasperation. Maggie interrupted the chaos with concern.

"Karina's alright, isn't she Jane? Everything worked out ok, didn't it?"

"Oh yeah. Turns out that was the best day of my life. Mama was shocked, but everything turned out alright. I had preeclampsia and my blood pressure got really high. I think I knew all along, but didn't want to say, you know?"

"Oh for heaven's sake. I can't, I can't even," said my receptionist, red-faced and wiping the tears from her eyes.

"Hey, I was always a big girl," Jane tried to explain. My receptionist exploded into another fit of breathless giggles and we couldn't help but smile watching her.

Maggie said, "Jane, I'm so glad that you and Karina are alright. I want a big family, so I know how important she is to you."

"You're doing things the right way, honey. You go to school. You get a career. A nice guy will come along. I did everything backassward," Jane said. The group had resumed eating. Jane, the "I didn't know I was pregnant" healthcare worker seemed an unlikely advice columnist, but Maggie was listening quite attentively. At this point, it was just Maggie and Jane going back and forth with question and answer.

"So you never wanted to marry?" Maggie asked.

"Didn't have no time for a man. I had a new baby and I needed to finish school. I had Karina to think of," Jane answered matter-of-factly.

"You did an amazing job with her," Maggie said. We all knew that Karina would be going off to college in the fall and that Jane was saving to help her with tuition. We took turns giving Jane a lift to the bus stop because her "car allowance" was going towards her daughter's college fund.

"I admire your courage," Maggie said.

"Well thanks darlin'. But sometimes you just do what you gotta do. Enough about me. How are things with you? How are those applications?"

"Oh, they're coming," she answered.

"You don't give up now. Karina tells me all the time that her studies are hard and that some kids have more time to go out because they don't give one-hundred percent at school."

"What do you tell her?" Maggie asked, genuinely interested. The rest of us had tuned out by now. I was watching Maggie watch Jane.

"I tell her that's bullshit. I tell her to get her lazy self back in her room to study. Then I tell her I love her and that she's the best thing that ever happened to me."

"Sounds good," Maggie said smiling.

"Remember, baby. Eye on the prize," Jane concluded, dipping her last fry in the little plastic tub of barbecue sauce.

Maggie was quiet as she repackaged her Tupperware set into its carrying case. I could tell that she'd grown pensive, but in good faith, we had a busy afternoon ahead and there was no more time for questions. Also, no matter how close we'd grown, some stones were best left unturned and I wasn't polite enough to ask questions out of obligation. We vacated the lunchroom table and returned to our stations, each of us our island, silently breezing past the others through narrow corridors.

Months passed. The winter was mild and summertime weather seemed to usurp the spring. The gang had taken to eating lunch outside at times, and I had heard Maggie mentioning to some of the other ladies that Joe was feeling tired lately and wasn't eager to go out much.

"He was dating this gal from his work, so I figured that's why he didn't want to hang out. You know it can be weird when you have a friend who's a girl," Maggie explained.

"You got that right," the serial monogamist chimed in.

"He said that he has no energy," Maggie noted.

"That doesn't sound right. Maybe he should come in for an appointment," another lady suggested.

"Yeah, maybe he needs blood work or something," offered another staffer.

"I called him the other day and he said that things weren't really working out with his new girlfriend, so they broke it off. I asked him if he wanted to catch a movie to take his mind off things. I was sure he was going to say yes, but then he said he was too tired to go out."

"Maybe he's depressed," suggested a receptionist.

"Maybe," mused Maggie not believing that explanation.

"Trust your gut, honey," said Jane. "If it doesn't seem right, it's not right."

Maggie forced a smile and said, "Thanks guys. I'll talk to Joe about coming in for an appointment. You know how boys can be. " We wrapped up with some idle banter about the benefits of having a deep fryer at home and an informal poll on who had ever eaten a chocolate-covered Twinkie. Maggie was quiet and seemed to be lost in her own thoughts until the rustle of plastic plates and forks returned her to the moment as we cleaned up around her.

The following Wednesday Maggie clutched a chart to her chest and plopped down on the chair in my office. I was sitting at my desk, shuffling through paperwork in between patients.

"The 11:30 a.m. just cancelled so we have a few minutes," she said.

"Great!" I closed the chart I'd been looking at and put it aside. "So, what's going on? Anything?"

"Well, a lot maybe."

"Sounds decisive." I reached across the desk to retrieve the 11:30 a.m. patient chart she was holding. With her hands now free, she nervously picked at her cuticles. "What's wrong, Mag?" I asked, putting my pen down so she'd know that she had my undivided attention.

"You know how last week we were all talking about how Joe's been tired?"

"Sure, I remember."

"Well, even before he started getting tired, I started asking myself whether this was right."

"Whether what was right?"

"Whether my path is right. Whether my friends are okay. Why I'm doing what I'm doing."

"This is all very existential for 11:30 in the morning," I said, trying to lighten the mood.

"Remember when Jane was talking about Karina at lunch?"

"Yes and the surprise birth."

"Yes," she chuckled, "Well, I started thinking about my life and balance, you know. I'm neither here nor there. I'm not married. I don't have kids. I don't have my career in order. And a friend who has always been so solid and so stable in my life seems to be slipping away."

"Let's start with the easy stuff. Joe is not slipping away. Maybe he's just tired, or maybe he is just bummed out that he and his girlfriend didn't work out. All the more reason he should come in for an appointment. Somewhere at least, if not here."

"You're right."

"And maybe he's not tired. Maybe the friendship is changing for him. Maybe you thought he was a friend for a lifetime and he's really going to be a friend for a season. You can't change that. You're just going to have to live it and see."

"I know that's true, but I wish I knew the outcome."

"You don't, really. Life would be too boring if you did. As for marriage and kids, your time will come, and to quote a very wise phlebotomist we both know, 'Don't do it backassward.'" Maggie laughed and her posture seemed to relax a bit.

"And how about your career? Are you having second thoughts about medical school?"

"I don't know. I don't think so, but I've realized that you can over intellectualize anything and I hope I didn't do that here. I hope I didn't enter the medical field because that's all I know."

At first I didn't know what she meant, but then I remembered that her father was a practicing OB/GYN. She appeared to become physically ill and I knew that all of these concerns had been eating at her for a while. Voicing her feelings aloud had somehow made them real.

"Okay, now don't panic. There's nothing you can't recover from. If you're uncertain about your career, then you need to figure out why and once you've figured out why, if the only solution is to change direction, then that's what you must do. If you're uncertain about your friendship, then all you can do is be supportive and know that you'll have no regrets."

"I know you're right, I guess so... Hold on a minute, my butt is buzzing." She reached into her back scrub pant pocket and pulled out her cell phone.

"Hi. Yes. Well, what's going on? Umm, ok. Hold on a minute." She placed the phone down on her lap and said, "This is Joe. He said that he really doesn't feel great and thinks that maybe he should come in for some blood work or something."

"Tell him to come now. We have a cancellation. Let's just get to the root of this."

"Can you come now? Ok, come right over. Ok, see you soon." She said and hung up the cell. "Thanks for everything. To be continued, huh?"

"To be continued," I said, and she got up to go in the back to make some patient calls and tidy up the exam room before Joe arrived. After a whispered exchange in the lobby, Maggie brought Joe back. You could see the worry on her face and it seemed like weeks had elapsed since our earlier conversation. She handed me his chart and said that he'd lost five pounds, but he hadn't been eating much.

"I'm nervous," she said with her eyes brimming with tears.

"Don't be," I answered. "Strong, young men usually don't have anything seriously wrong. Let's see what we find and then we can take things one step at a time." She sat down at her desk to make some patient calls, and I headed into the exam room with Joe.

"Well, we meet again. I'm sorry you haven't been feeling well," I said.

"Hi, doctor. I know. Me too. It's good to see you again," he said, rising out of his seat to shake my hand.

"You, too. So what's been going on?" I half expected him to dance around a bit and then launch into a monologue about how he was depressed about his recent relationship, but he didn't.

With eerie seriousness, he said,

"I know something's wrong. I've been tired—really tired. And I have no appetite. That's why I've lost a few pounds."

"Have you been unusually stressed about anything? Has anything changed?"

"No. Everything's fine. I like my job. I'm just so tired and I get full easily."

"Any reflux symptoms? Sour taste in your mouth? Fullness in your throat? Trouble swallowing? Burping? Belching? That sort of thing?"

"Not really. I guess I get a little indigestion here and there, but nothing out of the ordinary. Sometimes I have a hard time breathing when I lie flat at night, but I figured that I was eating too late and going to bed on a full stomach, so I cut out nighttime snacks."

"Any lumps, bumps, changes in your skin?"

He hesitated and said, "No. Well, I'm not sure."

"What does that mean?"

"It's probably nothing, but I appreciate you seeing me today."

So polite, I thought to myself, *even in spite of his feeling lousy and his mounting concern.*

"I can't tell if I have a lump under my armpit," he finally said.

"Okay, let's start with some blood work and then I want to do an exam. Here's the gown. Open to the front like a coat and take everything off except your underwear," I said, reaching for the doorknob.

"OK," he muttered and started getting undressed.

Maggie was there when I left the exam room.

"How is he?" she asked almost holding her breathe while incessantly tapping her foot.

"Maggie, we just talked. I haven't even examined him yet. I'll send Jane in to draw his blood, and we'll all talk once we're finished."

"OK," she sighed and turned away.

Joe was perched on the exam table, reinforcing his Band-aid from the blood draw when I reentered. Wisps of blond hair fell boyishly over his forehead and his cheeks pinked up in anticipation of the physical exam. He was bashful, but more strikingly, he was concerned. He was worried in a raw and frightened way. That kind of worry is contagious. Although we are taught to maintain a healthy doctor-patient distance in the interest of objectivity, fear can narrow that space. Fear of the unknown is the great equalizer. I methodically worked my way from the top down starting with the head and neck exam.

"Are these glands sore?" I asked with my hands below his chin, my fingertips abutting his thyroid gland. "Swallow for me." Joe, ever dutiful, allowed me to seesaw him through sitting, lying, and more sitting maneuvers as he answered my questions.

"I know that you mentioned something under your armpit. Don't show me, ok? I want to see if I can reproduce the finding."

"Ok."

I tried to provide reassurance even as I discovered the painless axillary mass. To this day, I am uncertain if he knew all along and was strangely relieved that I validated his suspicion or had no idea and was just happy to have a potential explanation for his symptoms. It was one p.m. on a Wednesday afternoon and by 2:45 p.m. he was having his PET CT (a scan we traditionally order when we are concerned about malignancy) and by 4:30 p.m., we were back in the office discussing its implications.

Joe had asked Maggie to join him in the room as I delivered results. They sat across from my desk, defeated, quiet, and attentive. Although I had trouble seeing over the piles of paper and the cups of pens that landscaped the top of my desk, I noticed that Maggie was touching Joe's forearm. Ironically, Maggie was sitting in the very chair she'd sat in for her initial interview.

"I don't know how much the radiologist told you. I don't want to repeat anything," I began.

"Don't worry about that. You just tell me what you know," Joe said with not so much as a quiver in his voice.

"Well, the axillary mass we discovered during the physical exam was confirmed on ultrasound. The radiologist said that your PET CT is highly suspicious for malignancy in your lungs," I said trying not to avert my gaze. Moments like this demanded eye contact no matter how tempting eye-aversion might have been.

"So I have cancer," Joe said.

"It would seem likely. Yes. Things are pointing towards Hodgkin's Lymphoma but we'll need a lymph node excision and possibly a bone marrow biopsy to confirm it and stage the disease," I answered catching Maggie. Her eyes were brimming with grief.

Composed, but clearly shaken, Joe rose from the chair, extended his hand to me and expressed his gratitude for my speedy attention to his needs.

"Thank you again, Dr. Holt. I guess I'll wait to hear from you tomorrow?" he asked.

"Yes and don't eat or drink anything when you get up. I'm going to speak with a surgeon and an oncologist."

"OK. Thanks again."

I cleared the morning of appointments the next day, as I would need to make rapid-fire phone calls to oncologists, surgeons, and insurance carriers. Testing and appointments all required pre-certification numbers and the standard line for issuing pre-certification authorization was: "I'm sorry, but it can take up to seventy-two hours to get a pre-certification number."

I don't have to tell anyone how frustrating it is to hear someone in customer service read a scripted line off a cue card while you, the listener, are growing more panicked by the threat of delayed response and more impatient by the seeming nonchalance of the representative. Eventually though, pre-cert numbers were issued and paperwork was faxed, paving the way for Joe to access his tests and subspecialists all within the next forty-eight hours.

Joe went for his consultation with the surgeon in the morning and the oncologist in the afternoon the next day.

Further evaluation of his PET CT revealed lung involvement and, looking back, this could have explained his vague complaint of breathing difficulties while lying flat. Lymph node pathology confirmed Hodgkin's Lymphoma and his bone marrow biopsy was fortunately negative for the disease. Joe was diagnosed on a Wednesday and was discussing a treatment plan for his cancer by Friday night.

Maggie never worked in the office again. Joe was here alone, with family far away and Maggie quit her job to support him full time as he grew weaker from punishing chemotherapy sessions. Her faith in the process of life was inspiring. These were the cards her friend was dealt and she was going to help him play the hand in an honorable and decent way. Joe had always been there for her, and this was her chance to reciprocate. I never saw Maggie or Joe again, although we did correspond for a while.

Joe became, for a brief time, a shell of his former self as documented in the pictures he'd send from time to time. At first, you couldn't even tell that he'd lost his eyebrows because he was so fair, but the absence of lashes betrayed the chemotherapy patient every time. When we did speak by phone, I was struck by how resolute he was about his recovery. He'd say things like, "When this nightmare is over," or, "When I get back on my feet . . . " And he would end every conversation with gratitude, thanking me for seeing him that day and for orchestrating his early diagnosis and treatment. It was mind-numbing to me that he wasn't consumed with anger at the injustice of his circumstances or at least wrapped tightly in a blanket of self-pity. Joe was neither. He was poised, well mannered, and hopeful. I sent him a "Happy Anniversary" card each year for five years after his diagnosis to celebrate and commemorate his survival. To the best of my knowledge, he is doing well and is disease-free.

After Maggie evaporated from the office, I couldn't see much reason to stay. I rationalized that I had gleaned from this job experience more than I'd hoped, and I gave my notice. I worked for the next three months without Maggie and with my sights set on a new beginning.

***

I have told this story a number of times when I've given speeches about primary care medicine and about the importance of physician advocacy in complex care cases. At the end of the talk, the most frequently asked question has always been:

"Did Maggie and Joe ever become a couple?"

And would you believe that it is usually a man in the audience who asks? Let it be known that there still are some hopeless romantics out there.

Maggie and Joe did not become a couple, but they did stay friends for a lifetime. Joe regained his health and re-embraced his future and his life and Maggie continued on with her schooling, pursuing her professional dreams and re-establishing, in her own mind, what she wanted out of her career and her personal life.

This experience taught me two things: there's nothing you can't recover from; and you need a doctor when you're well, not when you're sick. Living the experience gave me the courage to pursue a career as a solo practitioner and reshaped my own perception of what a primary care doctor should be—not only a good diagnostician, but a fierce patient advocate. When I initially opened my practice, I gave neighborhood talks on healthcare topics and doctor-patient experiences. I could never stomach those cheesy ads with doctors posing stiffly with over-whitened, slightly constipated smiles and arms folded firmed across their chests. I vowed that I would never advertise the practice, so I gave talks as a way to introduce the office to the neighborhood.

When I speak about this experience, the talk is titled: "You need a doctor when you're well, not when you're sick." Had Joe not had an established relationship with a physician and had he not had easy access to her, the initial diagnosis would certainly have been delayed. And had he not had physician advocacy slicing through the mire of insurance company red tape and regulations, his treatment plans would certainly have been muddied. A pre-established doctor-patient relationship was the lens through which to see clearly his whirlwind forty-eight hours from diagnosis to treatment initiation. Sick, despairing people are often not the most discriminating, so I wouldn't advise waiting until you don't feel well to find a physician. Ironically, we are all under the opposite impression: we go to the doctor when we're sick, not when we're well.

Sparing mortal injury or terminal illness, there's nothing you can't recover from. If we all had such faith in our ability to restore ourselves, calculated risk-taking would be less scary. Approaching a pretty girl would be more tangible for the young man with a great sense of humor and coke-bottle glasses. The accountant with a great singing voice might audition for that job at a piano bar even though it seems like an "unsafe" choice. I could philosophize forever about how our insecurities and lack of faith sabotage our potentials. But perhaps with this insight, just before we talk ourselves out of a new opportunity, we can take a moment to say instead, "There's nothing I can't recover from."

Chapter Two

LIFE PERMITS U-TURNS

When you think about your life
About the you you'd like to be
I hope that you can find your heart
In both work and play, you'll see.

If your work is like a calling
Like an ocean's wave mid-swell
Then it won't seem like a job at all
Up and forward you'll propel.

Disentangle from the shackles
The confinement of the "shoulds"
Focus your attentions
On the options of the "coulds."

In the words of William Shakespeare,
"To thine own self be true."
These words—easier to read than live
Expectations cloud your view.

I believe that you alone can know
What's really at your core
People pleasing—chasing praise
Your true self this will obscure.

Life permits us to make U-turns
In search of your true light
The path may not be straight
With honest steps, it will be right.

***

He came into the lobby, unsnapping his helmet while holding the door open for his passenger. Her helmet was still on when she walked in, and she turned away from the check-in counter to find a seat in the lobby. Once seated, she fiddled with the chinstrap and unzipped her jacket. He approached the check-in counter to register and to sign in for his new patient appointment.

He was instantly likeable. His short, cropped hair and big, innocent, brown eyes didn't seem to belong under a motorcycle helmet. The receptionist requested his insurance card and any medical records he might want copied, asking,

"How are you doing today?"

"Fine, thanks. How are you? By the way, I'm Tommy. It's nice to meet you."

"Nice to meet you, Tommy," she answered. "I'll prepare a chart for you and get you back shortly." Reception positions in a doctor's office can be virtual firing squads for surly, short-tempered patients. Don't get me wrong. Most of my patient experiences are exceedingly pleasant, but any recalcitrance has been diluted first by the receptionist and then by the nurse before a patient gets to me. So all of the office front linesmen really soften the blow. Fortunately, Tommy was an easy patient.

"Thanks. Take your time," he said, finding a seat by his passenger.

Just as the receptionist looked down to complete her work, his lady friend unfastened her helmet to reveal a bowl of curly, gray hair. They'd taken a far corner seat in a spacious lobby. Between the distance from the check-in counter and the ambient sound of the radio, their conversation was muffled. The nurse appeared, holding the prepared chart and looked around the lobby to locate the next patient.

She whispered to the receptionist, "Who's he with?" Raised eyebrows and a silent shoulder shrug confirmed that she hadn't figured it out either.

The nurse beckoned, "Tommy, welcome. Come on back." After he was roomed and vitals were taken, the nurse handed me the chart, editorializing, "He's a nice boy."

I recognized the last name and wondered if there was any relation to a woman in my practice who shared the name. Due to the ever expanding, exceedingly complicated privacy rules that govern medicine nowadays, I couldn't come out and just ask. I would have to wait and see what unfolded during our doctor-patient interview.

"So, Tommy, I see you've just had a birthday. Happy twenty-sixth," I said.

"Oh, yes. Thanks."

"Let me ask you a few questions before we tune you up."

"Sounds good," he said with a smile.

"So, any surgeries? Tonsils? Appendix?"

"Tonsils out as a kid," he said.

"Anything new? Improved upon? Exchanged for something better?" I joked.

"No. All the parts are the same. No changes," he laughed.

He was a nice boy. *His easy smile and welcoming manner will serve him well*, I thought to myself.

"How about your family history?" I asked. "Are your parents living?"

"Yes, both."

"Generally healthy?"

"Yes, they're both well. In their fifties. You know my mom, Gloria."

"Oh, of course," I acknowledged. So this *was* the same family. His mother had established as a patient a few years earlier. Gloria was a well woman with fortunately few health ailments so she had spent some time during the office visit beaming about her children. Her daughter had met and married a man from Texas during her pediatric residency and had stayed out there, much to her mother's chagrin. And Tommy had recently been transferred to Australia for a work project, but his tour there was coming to a close and he'd be closer to home again soon.

"So, you're the son who's just returned from Australia."

"That's me." His tan cheeks picked up the faintest pink hue. Skin his color didn't show a blush much, but if you looked closely it was there.

"Mother's pride and joy," I needled. "I've heard a lot of nice things about you. Welcome back."

"Thanks."

"Didn't your mother tell me you'd be getting married soon?" I asked, testing my own memory of his mother's office visit.

"Yes. Almost six months from today as a matter of fact."

"How are the plans coming?"

"Coming along, I guess. My fiancée and her mother have really taken off and run with things. Once I saved for the ring, it seemed like my biggest job was done," he said.

"Fair enough." I reached for an exam gown and a lap drape, explaining that the opening is in the front. I stepped out so he could change and let him know that the nurse would be back to draw his blood.

"I'll be here," he said cheerfully as he examined the dressing gown, looking for the way into it.

The nurse exited the exam room with gloved hands inverting the newly filled tubes of blood. I went to take the chart back from her as she inserted the tubes into the centrifuge.

She held onto the chart and said, "You know he's engaged. He told me when I was drawing the blood. He said that he was a fainter, so I told him that we had to keep talking through the whole thing and that way it'd be over before he knew it," she asserted proudly. "Well, aren't you going to say anything?!"

"What do you want me to say? Congrats on the engagement? I'm glad he didn't faint? Good job on the blood draw?" I quipped.

"No!" the nurse responded with disgust. "Is he engaged to the lady who came in with him? She's more than twice his age!"

"Listen, this is not some daytime talk show. I just receive information; I don't dig for it. Besides, I didn't realize he came in with anyone. I never make it out to the lobby. Now give me the chart so I can get back in the exam room."

I left her in the lab, muttering to herself about the age difference between our love birds until the din of the turning centrifuge transformed every voice around it into white noise.

The physical exam was uneventful and he, like his mother, was of healthy stock. At the end of the visit, we were wrapping up with some suggestions about how to avoid razor burn, or folliculitis barbieri as it may be termed more clinically, when I asked a few more questions about the wedding.

"So, is your mother excited about your upcoming nuptials?"

"Oh mom. Yeah. You know she's pretty easygoing. She gets along well with Danielle. In fact, they have a lot in common." He answered. I couldn't help but wonder if their generation was one of the commonalities they shared.

"Where will you be getting married?" I asked.

"In Pennsylvania, closer to Danielle's hometown. Her family

is small, but they don't like to travel much, so my side will head out there."

"Well, Tommy, good luck with your planning," I said with one hand on the doorknob, ready to exit so he could change out of the exam gown.

"I will be back in a few months for an employee physical. The form requires a face-to-face encounter and I will need that to reenter my branch here in the States."

"Anytime. We will be looking forward to seeing you again and hearing about your plans. Say 'hi' to your mom for me," I answered.

"Will do," he smiled, hopping off the exam table.

I exited the room with the nurse mouthing to me silently, "So?"

"So?" I parroted back with exaggerated theatrics and raised my hands up in a show of defenselessness and I entered the next exam room. Tommy stopped at the checkout desk to settle his bill with motorcycle gear back in tow. After wishing the staff a good day, he turned to his lady friend and said "Gran, are you ready? We're all set."

She picked up her helmet from the seat beside her. Setting a magazine down on the lobby coffee table, she said, "Yep. I was just getting caught up on the latest gossip." He held the door open for her and allowed his grandmother to exit first. The nurse and receptionist picked their jaws up just in time to smile and wave to the couple telling them both to stay well. Once the door was securely closed, they looked at each other and laughed.

It was a few months before I saw any member of the family again. The next to visit the office was his mom.

"Gloria, you're looking a little tired. What's going on?" I asked. This kind of open-ended question is just what the medical business magazines instruct you not to ask. It's hard to keep the office visit to the six-minute maximum if your questions are open-ended. Then again, if I subscribed to this philosophy, I'd have no stories to tell.

Gloria answered, "Well, I'm here on my lunch hour because I think I have another one of those sinus infections. It seems like I get them this time of year."

Looking at my office visit flow sheet, I tell her that she's right. It was March last year when she had her last bout of sinusitis. "Maybe allergies contribute since this is happening in the springtime. Pop up on the exam table and let's look at you," I instructed, reaching for my otoscope. "How's everything else?"

"Oh, you know, busy. My job is crazy. Laying people off without replacing them, but there's no reduction in workload. And Tommy's wedding is approaching," she paused.

"Weddings spotlight family pathology," I observed. "There's always a moment when the couple thinks that it would be easier to head to Vegas and get married by an Elvis impersonator,.."

She chuckled weakly and broke into a paroxysmal coughing fit befitting her sinusitis and evolving bronchitis. "I know what you mean. Even Tommy seems a little distracted. You know how even-tempered he is, but lately he clams up if you ask him what's bothering him. He seems so easily irritated," she said.

"Wow, that doesn't seem like Tommy." I replaced the otoscope in its holder.

"I know. He's always been such a good boy. I don't know what to make of him seeming so upset. I ask him if he and Danielle are alright, and he always says they're fine. But he never elaborates."

I sit on my backless rolling stool and reach for my prescription pad. As I'm writing her antibiotic prescription, I say, "Like I said. Weddings are stressful. All you can do is offer to be his sounding board and be ready if he does come to you with anything."

"Oh, I'll be ready. And you know that Tommy is very close to my mother," she added.

"I believe that I do know this," I said, smiling to myself as I recalled the day my staff had Tommy riding off into the sunset to marry his grandmother.

"My husband, on the other hand, is not much of a talker. You've not met him. He doesn't go to doctors. He's stubborn like his own father was. He loves Tommy, but has always had some difficulty communicating with him. I guess he's the strong, silent type. My mom and I more than make up for it, huh? I don't want to keep you," she said apologetically, reaching for her bag.

"Not at all. I love hearing about your son and the upcoming wedding. Let me know if you don't feel better after taking the antibiotic."

"Will do." She headed toward the exit and I heard her wishing the rest of the staff a good day as she left.

It wasn't long 'til we heard from Tommy. I saw his name posted on the daily schedule, listing "work physical exam" as the nature of the visit. I assumed that he was back from Australia and reentering his branch in the States. I wouldn't bring the subject up, but I wondered to myself how the wedding plans were coming and whether he would divulge anything about what might be troubling him. He arrived alone this time, driving a sensible car. As always, he greeted the receptionist, asked how her day was going, and took a seat in the lobby. He fumbled in his bag for some medical forms so he could be ready to hand them to the nurse when she called him back.

The nurse handed me the chart and said, "No blood work needed for these forms, so I told him that I'll save my vampire trick for another time. Our boy's just not right today though. You'll see." She handed me the chart and directed me to the exam room where he was waiting. I hesitated for a moment. You never know what you're going to get behind door number one and I have been humbled enough times to know that there's no predicting how an office visit will evolve.

Tommy sat in the patient's chair next to the exam table. He

was dressed in jeans and a collared shirt. I always interview patients sitting in a regular armchair, dressed in their street clothes. I think this allows for a more open dialogue and puts us on an equal playing field. By the time patients are disrobed in a flimsy gown, specimenized on a higher than is comfortable exam table, they usually aren't interested in idle chit-chat.

"Hi, sir. Welcome back. That purple is a good color for you," I comment.

"Oh, thanks. Yeah. I'm back for that work physical I told you about."

"So you're here to stay then? No more Australia?"

"Here to stay," he assured me.

"Your mother must be thrilled. With the time difference and all, communicating with you in Australia probably got tough at times."

"It can be tricky, but everyone got pretty computer savvy. Even Gran got into email and Skype. It was funny. She'd keep wondering where the camera was and would get unnaturally close to it asking, 'Can you see me? Can you see me?' When in reality, her face was distorted like a fun house mirror."

I laughed.

"She cracks me up," he added, shaking his head.

I glance at the form and ask if I can rattle off some of the questions so that we can get through the mundane fact fill-ins.

"Any hospitalizations in the last five years?"

"No."

"Any prescription medications?"

"Nope."

"Any history of smoking? Cigarettes or otherwise?" I looked up.

"Nope. Never took a puff." My thought bubble read, *What a nice boy!*

"Any history of broken bones?"

"I had a wrist fracture when I was ten. I fell off a jungle gym at recess," he answered.

"Fair enough. I'll write that in. Certainly that's pertinent to how you'll perform your job in finance, right? Which wrist?"

"Left," he said after a moment's thought to jog his memory.

I quickly scanned the forms to make sure that we'd covered the pertinents and recapped my pen. "I think that covers the basics. The rest is cut and paste immunization record information after the physical exam notes. So, how is it to be back?"

"Great. Australia's a beautiful place. But culturally, I belong here. I'm kind of accustomed to a fast pace, and I like city living. I'm looking forward to saving up and getting a place in the city soon." He looked down and began mindlessly picking at his palms.

"How are the wedding plans coming along?" I asked.

"Fine. Like I said before, I'm out of the loop," he said, barely lifting his eyes off the industrial white tile.

"Fair enough. Let's do this cursory physical exam and get you back to work," I said, leaving the exam room so he could get unchanged. Upon my reentering, I found him head down, picking at his hands. "What are you trying to do? You're going to peel the whole epidermal layer of your skin off." I took his hands in mine, holding his palms up to display angry, scaling skin. "This has got to hurt," I remark.

"It does. It's making me crazy. I used to just get a little eczema with the change of seasons. Now I'm shedding like a reptile."

"Sometimes we see eczema like this with celiac sprue or food sensitivities. Any stomach troubles?"

"No, not really. My appetite's decreased, but that's because I have so much going on."

"No nausea, diarrhea, vomiting?" I ask looking at the weight chart.

"No. Nothing like that."

"You know, you're down eight pounds since I last saw you. You don't need to lose weight. You need five pounds to fight off a cold, right?"

"I know. I need to be more conscious of it. I'll try to watch more."

"We can't have the groom falling out of his tux now, can we? That would be quite a scene," I said, trying to lighten the mood. I turned back to him as I reached for the sink faucet.

"I'm not sure there's going to be a groom," he admitted, looking straight ahead as if he'd rehearsed saying this out loud, but he just wasn't sure to whom he'd be talking. I shut off the running water and dried my hands with my industrial-strength hand towelettes.

"Oh." I paused. "Are you sure?"

"I am," he said, still not to anyone in particular.

"Does Danielle know?"

"No."

"Does your mother know?"

"No."

"The wedding's in two months, right?" I ask.

"Seven weeks," he answered, like an inmate on death row would count down the days 'til his execution.

I was standing at the sink when I decided instead to take a seat in the armchair where the patients begin their initial interview. This seemed like a conversation that required sitting in a chair with a back; swiveling around on my doctor's stool didn't seem like the right posturing. These are the moments I dread a knock at the exam room door or an inopportune cell phone ring because so much hung in the silence. I was aware of the metronomic tick of the blue wall clock and equally aware that I seemed to be holding my breath. I exhaled and tried to casually take a big breath in like a swimmer might, careful not to make a sigh out loud or give the impression that I was disinterested in any way.

"You know, if you're sure, you'll need to tell them."

"I know," he said despairingly.

"Tommy, life permits U-turns. You wouldn't be the first person to call off a wedding. I myself have a few friends who needed to break their engagements. I'm sure it was devastating at the time, but no more devastating than entering into a marriage you feel is wrong. Hey, I'm not a shrink, but that's my two cents." The beauty of being an internist is the ability to use the disclaimer that "I am, in turn, not a therapist or psychiatrist."

"I wasn't going to bring anything up today. I didn't plan to say anything," he said, unfixing his eyes from their target on the striped wall and meeting my gaze.

"Well, this is as safe a place as any to say something. I capped my pen, which meant that nothing gets written in the chart. Do you want me to let you get changed? Are you okay perched on that exam table?" I asked.

"Yeah I'm fine. Sitting up here is the least of my problems," he said, shaking his head.

"Do you know what you're going to do? Do you know what changed?"

"Which answer do you want first?"

An amateur move executed on my part. No self-respecting therapist would ask two questions in succession, leaving no room for an answer in between. It was a good thing I was only an internist and was excused these indiscretions by my patients.

"I'll take any answer you're offering." I smiled.

He seemed relieved by this response and evidently wanted to keep talking. "I've got to tell everybody. I've got to call it off. I've known for months. I just keep finding excuses."

"You'll do it. You'll do the right thing," I reassured. "And how about part two? Do you know what changed? Or is that too heavy a question? Sometimes if you know why, it's easier to explain to people".

"Yeah," he chortled, "maybe not in this case."

"Ok," I said and fumbled with my pen, fighting the temptation to disrupt the silence with a meaningless platitude. Rubbing his eyes and running his fingers through his hair, he said, "When I was in Australia, I met someone."

"Hmm. That's an issue. Are you still in touch with this person?"

"Yes," he exhaled.

"Is she back in Australia?"

He looked right at me and said, "She's a 'he' and he lives here. I'm gay."

My thought bubble read, *oh crap*, but I said out loud, "Well, that's a U-turn, alright." He laughed heartily and fell back on the exam table with his bent legs swinging as if he were sitting at the edge of a dock. "Listen, I can't continue this heavy conversation with you on that perch with a Johnny coat cinched around your waist. I'm going to leave you to your thoughts. You get dressed and I'm coming back in two minutes," I said as I exited the room.

In the hallway, I shook my head, humbled again at being surprised by the twists and turns of an office visit. I ping-pong to the other exam room to see the next patient as Tommy changed. I picked up the chart to see what the chief complaint was: urinary tract infection. The nurse had already analyzed the urine with a color dipstick. Breathing a sigh of relief, I said to myself, "*This should be easy to address as long as I keep the open-ended questions to a minimum.*" It was nice to see this young woman with no urgent issues but her urinary complaints, and she left promptly with a prescription in her hand.

By that time, Tommy was dressed and I was ready to reenter the room and the conversation. His exam gown lay crumpled on the white exam-table paper much like a snake's skin might hold the shape of its former self once shed. I'm sure Tommy wished a simple disrobing was all that was needed to reveal his true self, but he knew the next steps were fraught with layers of complexity. Calling off the wedding and informing all of the guests of their newly liberated social calendar seemed like the least of his concerns. Invariably, he'd have to answer the "why?" question—at least for Danielle and his family. Somehow, he envisioned it being easiest to tell Danielle. Sure, she would drudge through the five stages of grief on her way to recovery— denial, anger, bargaining, depression, and finally acceptance— but he had every faith that she'd be ok in the end. She was a great girl, and once she learned to share herself again and once she regained faith in her instincts, she'd be ok.

His greatest trepidation was telling his family—namely his mother and father. He felt particular pressure, likely self-imposed, to bring joy and pride to his family. He and his sister, after all, were the hope and future of their parents. Tommy explained to me that his dad was a devoted family man and a dedicated provider, but was for all intents and purposes a bit emotionally distant. I remembered his mother insinuating this to me before, so the characterization of his dad as sidelined and stern did not come as a surprise to me.

"How will you tell them?" I asked.

"I guess just like I did here. I have to tell them I'm calling off the wedding, and I have to tell them why. Really, I've rehearsed this moment in my head a hundred times. I just haven't had the guts to go through with it until now."

I gathered my business card in addition to the cards of two counselor colleagues of mine. (The real psychologist types who intentionally ask open-ended questions.)

"Here's my business card. You can reach me anytime. And here are two folks' names and numbers who might be helpful either to you or to your parents," I said, handing him the cards.

He looked contemplatively at the cards. "Thanks. I'm definitely going to hold onto these. My mom may want to talk to someone. This will be hard for her, I think."

"Listen. As an outside observer, I can tell you that your mother adores you. You are her pride and joy. Agreed, this is probably not how she envisioned the future—not your future and not her future—but she adores you. And she should because you're a good egg."

He nodded and I continued, "You better hang onto that because that's as close as I get to a compliment. I can't risk your head getting so big that you can't get out of here. You've got stuff to do after all." I smiled at him then, and he smiled with me.

"Yeah I've got stuff to do alright," he nodded and gathered his things to go.

"Please have your mother call if I can help at all. Remember," I said, patting him on the shoulder about to open the exam room door to see him out, "life permits U-turns. Just be honest with yourself and with them and things are going to work out ok. It may take a while, but everything's going to be ok."

"Thanks. And mom may call. She may not even need the phone cause you'll hear her screaming from our house ten miles away." I was happy to see his sense of humor returning.

"Good luck, Tommy. Now get out of here. Call if you need, and I'll get those papers in by the end of the week."

"I will and thanks," he said and wished the staff a good day on the way out.

"Good luck with the wedding," the receptionist shouted as she waved goodbye. I cringed as I overheard this from the hallway heading to my back office. My thought bubble read: *If you only knew . . .*

It wasn't long before we heard from Gloria. I saw her on the daily schedule with the office visit marked: discuss a few things. The nurse was quick to point out that she didn't know what form I wanted for the visit.

"Do you want a progress note or a physical exam form?" she

asked, clearly disturbed that the vagueness of the complaint was derailing her chart preparations.

"How about the 'discuss a few things and I don't want to tell the medial receptionist the nature of the visit' form," I quipped back.

Those blue eyes rolled up at me in feigned annoyance. "Just for that smartass response, I'm going to use a progress note form. I hope you like that," she humphed and paper-clipped the form to the chart with exaggerated effort. Those of you who are married to a P.C. and a keyboard may be cringing at my reference to a paper chart, but they are still in use. Don't tell anyone.

Gloria was roomed uneventfully with no unsolicited nursing commentary, which I found odd. *She's one cool cucumber,* I thought to myself, if she didn't send any distress signals off to the nurse. Of course, the nurse could have been having an off day herself and may have been less perceptive than usual. As I gathered my stethoscope and prescription pad and picked up the chart to enter the exam room, an unsettling thought occurred to me: *Maybe she doesn't know?* If that was the case, how would I begin? "Hi Gloria, what's new?" or "Hi Gloria, anything exciting happening?" I decided I would proceed as is always best: staying neutral and trying not to appear rushed.

I entered and extended my newly washed hand for a shake.

"Hi Gloria, it's good to see you," I started.

"Well, I wish I could say the same. I mean, it's always good to see you. It's just I didn't think I'd be back in here so soon," she lamented.

"Well, we're happy to have you. What's up?" That was the right open-ended question to launch, like a confession-seeking missile. Poor Gloria broke down in tears which evolved into sobs, and I gestured towards the tissue box on the end table.

"I purposely wore waterproof mascara despite the fact that I promised myself I wasn't going to cry. I've been crying for three weeks, and I'm not sure it's getting me anywhere. Tommy said you knew. He suggested I come in and get some guidance on where to go from here," she said with a nose blow and a decent pitch of the dirty tissue into the waste paper basket.

"Well, Gloria, I'm no expert, but you're probably doing some grieving—grieving the loss of who you thought Tommy was and grieving the loss of what you thought your future as a family would look like," I commented.

"Yes, I'm sure that's it. You know, I'm just so surprised. I can't believe that I didn't have a clue. I feel like such a fool. I've run memories of his growing up in my head over and over again. I didn't see any signs. He played little league baseball. He was on the debate team. He went to proms . . . "

My thought bubble read: *What the hell did the debate team have to do with anything?* But I cut the lady some slack. She was dealing with a lot after all.

"Was it something that I did? Was it because his father was distant?" she asked, reaching for an explanation.

"I can't say that I know much, but what I know for sure is that it was nothing that you did or didn't do and it has nothing to do with your husband's parenting style," I affirmed.

"I know you're right. I just am having trouble wrapping my head around this. I don't want his life to be hard, you know? You always want life to be easier for your kids and his life might be harder."

"Yes and no. Yes, it's harder to live the way a minority of the world lives. And yes, it's harder to live among people who could be judgmental or unaccepting. But isn't it harder to live a lie? Always looking over your shoulder hoping people don't suspect who you really are? Living fraudulently seems to be a much harder reality," I postulated. You never know what words might really stick with people. You throw your thoughts or ideas out there and it's always a bit of a crapshoot which ones might take.

But I could tell by the way her facial features started to relax that something in the dialogue helped. Something clicked for her.

"So you don't think it had anything to do with the fact that Tommy was particularly close to me and my mother growing up?" she asked, almost sheepishly. Before I could answer she interjected, "I don't mean to sound ignorant. It's just that you hear so many things. You take to the Internet and read some pretty crazy theories, you know?"

Thought Bubble: *Note to self: If my daughter comes out to me as gay in her young adulthood, I will not Google "parental responses to their newly affirmed gay children."* It sounded like much of the Internet dialogue was poorly researched and dangerously uncensored, but as I've come to find out in my career that particular characterization of the Internet is not unique to this subject matter.

"Listen," I said, "I'm not going to win a parent of the year award or anything but what I *do* know on this subject is what patients themselves have shared with me. These people have no reason to lie or misguide me. So, I feel like I know a little to the extent that my sources are authentic and real. If I can ventriloquize the words of another, I hope that I can shed some clarity. And later, when you're ready, you can always ask Tommy if what I said sounds right," I said.

"Sounds good. I really need all of the clarity I can get right about now."

"Every gay man or woman I've ever cared for who has elected to share his or her story of self-discovery with me has assured me that sexual orientation was in his or her wiring from very early on and not determined by any event, relationship, or circumstance that occurred in life," I stated somewhat matter-of-factly.

"I know that's right. I believe that too. It's just there are so many people who don't acknowledge that as true," she said despairingly.

"I just don't think that we can concern ourselves with misinformed Internet bloggers. Don't get me wrong, the Internet is a great thing and a wonderful way to disseminate a lot of powerful information, but unfortunately there's a lot of unregulated dialogue and everything written down is not founded in truth. We have been cultured to believe that the written word should be ascribed greater significance and meaning because it's written. Unfortunately, we have to change our perceptions," I lamented.

"I know. I need to stop seeking reassurance and have faith in what I believe. I yo-yo between acceptance and despair. I tell myself to be grateful that I have a happy, healthy, loving son and that works to console me for a while. Then I grieve the loss of the son I thought I had and start worrying about his life, his safety, his choices and I feel sick to my stomach again. I'm really a wreck." She started to well up with tears again.

"I think you're doing great. It's a lot to take in and you're being the graceful, bright woman I've always seen you be," I reassured, smiled, and asked, "How is your husband handling things?"

"You mean before or after he broke his mother's vase with a flying candlestick?" she asked facetiously.

"Oh, not that well then?"

"Things are better now. He is uncomfortable showing emotion and things were pretty raw there for a while. He apologized already to Tommy for some of the things he said. I know that he loves his son, and I know that he's going to come around in his own time,.."

"So no one's in danger? The home is safe?" I asked, hoping that her answer would be a convincing "no" and "yes" respectively because I didn't know what my obligation as a medical professional was if she suggested otherwise.

"Everyone is fine. Really," she said definitively.

We wrapped up the office visit with her agreeing that

speaking to a professional listener might be her next recourse. She left holding the same business cards her son held weeks ago as he exited the office.

"Now if you reach out to these folks, feel free to use my name to start the conversation. None of these therapists have reception staff, so they'll get their own phones," I advised.

The office visit was over. Gloria got up to leave and a handshake didn't seem like the right way to punctuate the experience. Wordlessly, she got up and extended her arms for a hug. Of course I did the same and she thanked me for listening and I thanked her for sharing her son and her life with me. I couldn't help but wonder if my third-year medical school preceptor who conducted mock patient-doctor interviews with us would have approved of our hug goodbye.

It would be three years until I'd see Gloria again. In that time, Tommy had requested a medical records transfer to a doctor in the city. Because that kind of request has to be done in writing, he had the opportunity to update me on his life. He'd called off the wedding and was back working at his old company and received that city transfer he'd wanted. He was excited about the move and thanked me for everything. His records were copied and sent out and the original chart was now dismantled and stored "in the back—a seldom entered room warehousing the stories of "inactive" patients.

Gloria's name appeared on the schedule next to CPE— complete physical exam. I was excited to see her and hoped that the last three years had treated her well. I entered the exam room saying, "Well, look who it is?" I extended my hand and she stood to give me a kiss on the cheek. "You look great."

"And so do you. It's great to see you again," she said.

"Ditto," I said, taking my seat on the backless, rolling stool. "I hope you're well. I'm glad we're seeing you for a physical exam. Are you feeling ok?"

"I'm great. No complaints. I'm overdue for a check-up. I haven't seen a doctor since the last time I was here."

"That was three years ago," I remarked. "I'm glad you've been so well."

"I've made a trip or two to employee health for sinus stuff, but in general, I can't complain," she said, looking around for wood to knock on. She settled for the armrest of the chair she was sitting in and rapped on it with her knuckles.

After itinerizing the routine preventative care tests she was overdue for—namely mammogram, pap smear, colonoscopy—I asked about the family.

"Is your mother still well?" I asked.

"Oh, yes. She's like the energizer bunny. Lives alone. Takes care of herself. And she's still close to Tommy."

"Oh good. I'm glad to hear that."

"In fact, my mother didn't blink an eye during that whole terrible time when Tommy was calling off the wedding. She was a great source of support to Tommy and to me and my husband."

"Good. I'm glad. And your husband is well?" I asked.

"Yes, he's fine. He's still not one for doctors but he's fine. And he and Tommy have come to a place of peace in their relationship."

"Wonderful. It sounds like the whole family is in a good spot. I'm happy to hear it! And Tommy? I hope he's well."

"He's great. Working and living in the city like he always wanted. He's particularly busy now though with all the planning," she said, baiting me for more questions.

I furrowed my brow and asked, "Planning? What's he planning?"

"A wedding," she answered. "He's met someone. His partner is very nice. Smart and ambitious with a good sense of humor. My family will be there, but only my husband will attend from his side. I think that was a real turning point for him. My husband, I mean. He wants to support his son even though his family won't."

"Wow. What a difference a few years make, huh?"

"You *better* bring photos. I want to see this dashing crowd in their wedding best." I shake my head and remark, "Would you have ever predicted that we'd be here now talking about Tommy's wedding?"

"Never," she said, smiling. And she looked genuinely happy and relieved.

"Life permits U-turns," I said.

"It certainly does," she answered.

***

How did Tommy have the presence of mind to follow his heart when doing so would be distinctly unpopular? His self-awareness was tremendous and he ultimately spared himself and the people close to him a lifetime of fraudulent family photos and deceptive memories. "To thine own self be true." You can't just say it, you have to live it.

Conversely, it's pretty easy to say that you love unconditionally as a parent, but when called to the task, can you do it? We would all like to say "unequivocally yes," but is it that easy? I don't know who was more courageous—Tommy himself or his parents. So often, parents think of their children as extensions of themselves. This may be especially true now in the age of the helicopter parent and the over-exposed "photo journalism" of Facebook. If a mom conceives of her child as an extension of herself, wouldn't it be difficult to love that child unconditionally if the child was somehow distinctly different? If a mother was a professional dancer, lanky and lithe, and her daughter was built a little more like her husband—stocky and stout—does that bother that mother just a little bit? When that mom enrolls her daughter in ballet and realizes that her daughter additionally does not possess her own natural flexibility and leg extension, does she turn a blind eye? Does she grieve the disparity in their physiques and abilities? Or does she celebrate her daughter for being her daughter? We all know how we want to answer the question. But loving and accepting a child unconditionally is hard and is completely selfless.

To all those struggling with their identity or their future, I hope they know that the world will not stop spinning on its axis if things don't evolve as planned. And just when you think that you stand alone with your thoughts—panicked and afraid, there will be someone standing by you and that person will love you unconditionally. Although the ending was very storybook for my Tommy and Gloria family, the bearer of that unconditional love is not always a parent and not always a family member. Sometimes our families or extended families can be the most disappointing and the least supportive. The Tommy's of the world often get dropped from the Christmas card list and get mysteriously deleted from the "send-all" graduation party invitation. If that is the unfortunate truth, then so be it. It seems much more vital to be true to oneself than to add a perfunctory picture to the holiday card wall.

If I'm faced with the task of parenting selflessly (and all parents are), I hope that I can channel Gloria's strength and focus. Through it all, she stood by her son, fortifying the bond that I always saw between them.

No matter what your political, cultural, or religious views, we could all agree on a few things: be true to yourself, love your children unconditionally, and life permits U-turns. All three tenets are easier to read than to live by, but I'd suggest that we keep trying.

Chapter Three

ANYONE CAN MARRY . . .

Anyone can marry
If you set your sights real low
Believe me when I say
There's more than one who you will know

Who as they head toward thirty
Will hear tic tock, tic tock
That is the metronomic sound
Of the "Biologic Clock."

You'll spend your life creating
The best you that you can be
Don't throw it all away
For the sake of "Fertility."

It matters who you marry
The decision shapes your life
Don't take the first who turns your head
For your husband or your wife.

Think of what <u>you</u> want
Or what mark <u>you</u> want to make.
The one who walks on that path too
That is the spouse you'll take.

***

Marriage is a complicated business and whom you marry is unarguably the most life-changing decision you'll make. It would seem that our pervasive electronic communication systems would facilitate our mating options. Online dating services ostensibly have the potential to pair people seamlessly— right down to religion, hair color and annual income. Somehow, though, the chemistry of two people uniting not only with one another, but also with their existing families and friends is not always easy to cook up.

As a generalist, I have the opportunity to know multiple generations of a family and an in-law family. The complexity of those dynamics are unlikely to be captured in texts or emails and can't be neatly arranged like stamps in an album no matter how accurate the online profile.

I first met Amy in her pre-college physical exam office visit. Tall and lithe, with a boyish build, she sat slightly slumped in the exam chair, waiting to be questioned. This visit often marks the exit from the pediatrician and the young person's initiation into the world of adult medicine. Her mom, Jill, stood at five feet, ten inches slightly pear-shaped unlike her narrow-hipped daughter. Jill was in the exam room before I could intercept the nurse to remind her of my need to see these young people alone and not with the infantilizing presence of their loving parent. Too late. Amy's mom was a patient, too, after all and already was familiar with the office processes and staff. Jill's hair was growing back in coarse pleats after the chemotherapy, which we'd laughed about because it was pin-straight and couldn't hold a curl before treatment.

"So Amy, you'll be heading off to college in the fall?"

"Yes."

"Excited?"

A gassy smile and head nod led me to believe that it wasn't as bad as heading off to the electric chair, but wasn't as good as a day at Disney for a six year old. This mother in the room thing wasn't working and would certainly jeopardize any chance I had at a relationship with this young lady.

"Mom, why don't you tell me what you want me to know, and then we'll shoo you off into the lobby."

Being the loving and responsible mom she was, Jill opened a folder and handed me each paper announcing its contents while licking her index finger to get a grip on the next record of importance.

"Here are her immunization records. I believe that the college form requires those. And here are the pediatric records— mostly weights and growth charts, I think. I've already made copies of these so they're yours to keep. And here's something I typed up about our family history. You may have this from my file, but I thought I'd have one in Amy's as well.

"Thanks, Mom," I said as I reached for each new document in the mother-doctor relay of information. All the while Amy sat slightly stooped, tan legs extended, ankles crossed, and eyes averted, thinking about anything but the present.

"That's it?" I asked.

"That's it. Amy, do you need me for anything?" Jill asked almost pleadingly as she picked up her bag, preparing to head out to the lobby.

"Nope." Amy answered, raising her head up enough to shake it. Mom exited, the door closing behind her and I let enough footsteps pass until I heard the lobby door open and shut before

I made an attempt at a re-introduction.

"So, Amy, it's nice to meet you. Your mother has only good things to say about you and your brothers."

"Thanks." She sat up a bit in the straight-backed chair now.

"Are you excited about going off to college?"

"Mixed feelings, I suppose. It's time for me to go and I feel ok about leaving now that she's doing better."

"Of course, it's been a hard year—a scary one at that."

Amy wordlessly nodded in agreement and we ran through the family tree with her reminding me that she's the youngest of four with three older brothers, the third of whom was a senior in college this year. Doing the math, it'd been just Amy and her mom for the last three years.

"And you know my father died ten years ago at age fifty-two of a brain tumor."

"Yes, I knew that. I'm sorry. He was too young."

"Yep," with a brisk head nod of agreement.

The rest of the office visit was a success by any estimation. Fortunately, she was well and we shared a few laughs about local current events and recent prom dress fashions.

"So, Amy, are you dating anyone fabulous?" I asked.

"No."

"Not fabulous? Or not dating anyone?" I chortled.

She laughed back. "Not dating anyone."

"Who did you go to the prom with?" I had already known of her attendance because we had just debated the merits of a strapless versus the "so last year" one-shoulder design.

"I went with a bunch of girls. We split the limo and went together."

"Oh that's nice," I tepidly replied, not knowing whether it was customary to go to a prom with a group of friends. It had been a while since my prom days. "You go to an all girls school, right?"

"Right."

"Is that ok? Socially and all?"

"Oh yeah, it's fine. Everyone's nice." Just then, her phone began to "ribbit."

"I think there's a frog in your bag."

"No," she said with a smile, "just got a text message. I'll get it later."

We wrapped up the office visit with the usual platitudes and I handed her my business card, reassuring her to call the office should she ever need anything while she was away at school. She assured me she would and off she went. With long strides and pretty blonde hair swooshing behind her, she met her mom in the lobby to be gently grilled about the visit.

The next time I saw Jill, Amy's mother, in the office, was six months later and December was already upon us. She explained that Amy's college transition had gone well and she had accumulated enough credits in high school to graduate from college in three years. She was already planning to schedule her spring semester classes on Tuesday, Wednesday, and Thursday to allow her four-day weekends at home. Jill's hair had grown in nicely and she fumbled with her newly found ringlet while saying that it would be nice to have Amy home again.

This office visit was for atypical chest pain. Jill had had chest wall radiation for breast cancer and was experiencing palpitations and chest discomfort, especially at night and at rest. After a thorough evaluation and conclusions drawn about what the cause was *not*, we narrowed down what the cause could be.

"Is this the same time last year that you had palpitations?" I asked glancing at the flow sheet in the chart itemizing office visit dates and the nature of the visit. "I believe we did a full cardiac workup at that time?"

"Yes, I think it was and, short of an autopsy, I think I've had just about every test," Jill answered.

"Is there something about December? Is there something about this season?"

"December seventh is the anniversary of my husband's death. I think this may have something to do with it," she answered from her spot on the exam table, Johnny coat tied at the neck with her feet touching the footrest. Shorter patients swing their legs nervously missing the footrests altogether, but Jill's well-pedicured feet stuck fast.

"Oh, I'm sorry."

"It's more complicated than it seems. Did I ever tell you that I was planning to leave him before he got sick? Our marriage was arranged. The two families knew each other and thought we'd make a good pair. And we did for a while and we had four beautiful kids to show for it. I was just getting my nerve up to ask him for a divorce when I got a call that he had had a seizure on the job site and was rushed to the local hospital. The whole year was a blur after that. By the next day, we knew about the GBM (glioblastoma multiforme) and by the day after that, we knew that it was inoperable. What was I to do then? We brought him home and I became a young widow."

"That must have been awful," I said. It's interesting the turn a "chest pain" office visit can take if you allow it. "Do you think the children suspected?"

"It's hard to know. Bob, my oldest, was already out of the house by then and the other three . . . I really don't know. I don't think so. Needless to say, I never spoke of my intentions or the fact that our marriage was arranged. It would have torn our families apart, and my decision would have been a great disappointment. I didn't need an exit strategy anymore and there was no reason for me to try to rewrite history. He died at home nine months after his diagnosis when Amy was just eight years old."

"I wonder if these palpitations could be the result of cumulative stressors. Maybe the upcoming holidays, your husband's passing, and this unresolved conflict—really this secret of sorts—are all contributing to these palpitations?" I suggested.

What a strong woman. I remarked to myself. She'd been a young widow, raised and supported four kids, and held onto a secret for decades. It couldn't have been easy. No wonder it was so nice that Amy would be spending more time at home. They'd become quite a team over the years.

The office visits between Jill and Amy ping-ponged back and forth over the years alternating between well visits and episodic sick visits. Each appointment provided an opportunity to catch up on their respective career, personal, and social lives. Amy ended up completing college in three years and pursuing a Master's degree in neuroscience at a local university.

Jill continued in remission and had grown accustomed to using a hair pick for her curls. Through Jill, I'd learned that her oldest son had relocated his family to Colorado for a job. Her second son was living the bachelor life in New York City and seemed enamored with nightlife and his job as a big-shot headhunter. Her third son had come out and was living with his partner also in New York City making a go of a career as a pet therapist.

During Amy's visits over the years, I'd heard about the trials and tribulations of graduate school and the "publish or perish" mantra of academics. She'd educated me on cruises she took and a recent trip to Dubai she'd taken with a newly engaged lady friend. The trip had been great and would probably nostalgically mark one of their last trips together as traveling companions. She had lived briefly on her own in a studio apartment, but for the purposes of cost containment, was now living with Jill again in the family home. Nine years had passed since our initial farewell to the pediatrician visit and Amy made an appointment for "neck pain," as it was noted on the schedule.

"Hi, Amy, what's new and exciting?"

"Not much exciting, but what's new is my neck. Namely the

pain in it."

She looked great. Honey-colored highlights framed her face and her hair was angled in an edgy cut. She remained tall and thin and seemed to have a penchant for ballet flats.

"What have you done? You're very tight in here," I said as I kneaded my thumbs into her sternocleidomastoid muscles.

Wincing, she answered, "If I knew, I wouldn't be here or at the very least I wouldn't keep doing it."

"How about your work station? Is it ergonomically sound? Are you on a computer a lot?"

"I don't know much about ergonomics, but I'm probably carrying a lot of tension in my neck. You know I worry about everything." This I had come to know. "Come to think of it, I have been on the computer more lately," Amy confessed.

"Oh, for work?"

"No, I joined some online dating sites. At first, a few of my friends did it as a lark and now it seems to be monopolizing a lot of my free time. When I'm not wearing some hideous cantaloupe-colored bridesmaid dress, I'm online seeing how many hits my profile has gotten."

Intrigued, I asked, "What kind of things did you write? Did you have to make any special requests?"

She said, "I want to meet a tall guy. I want my hand to look small resting next to his."

"Amy, being a small person myself, I don't claim to empathize with the importance of height in dating, but don't you think that there are other traits that could be more relationship-defining?"

"All I know is I'd like to wear heels," she replied dismissively, glancing down at her ballet flats.

"Fair enough. Just remember that you are a great girl with a lot more to offer than tall stature, right?" I admonished.

"Right."

I wrote her a prescription for Naprosyn and a muscle

relaxant. I recommended massage therapy telling her to take up Tai Chi as I handed her the prescriptions and directed her out.

Over the next few years, I didn't see much of Amy because she had moved in with her fiancé and was a forty-five-minute distance away now. Jill came in periodically and filled me in on the goings on of her family. After exchanging niceties and getting updates about the boys, I casually asked about Amy. Even if I didn't ask, the conversation would eventually circle back to Amy anyway because inevitably, Jill's concern for her would somehow relate to the office visit.

"How's everything, Jill?"

"Oh, alright. I was just wondering if I could have a few more of those anxiety pills. I don't use them a lot. You can see my last refill was over six months ago."

"Oh, I agree. You're not overusing these at all, and I'd be happy to refill them. I suppose the real question is, what anxiety are we medicating and is there any chance, we can eliminate the cause?"

Jill chuckled, "I think that eliminating the cause is called murder and is illegal. No, seriously, I'm worried about Amy. I know that she's almost thirty years old and needs to make her own decisions, but this relationship she's in has changed her interactions with me and with her brothers and even with her friends."

"Well, relationships *do* change family dynamics. Is it more concerning than that?" I put down my pen. There was nothing said here that needed to be documented in any medical record. I was careful to not reveal anything that Amy had ever said to me about her online dating. In fact, I was careful not to interject at all. It seemed important for Jill to relate her concerns in a forum where they wouldn't be refuted.

I learned that Amy and her fiancé lived in a nice apartment within reasonable commutable distance to their respective jobs.

Her fiancé was very orderly and kept things quite neat. It didn't sound like this fellow was alphabetizing cereal boxes, but Jill seemed a bit strained when speaking of his orderliness. I also learned that there were "house rules"—one of which was "no phone calls." He liked the apartment quiet at night after work and didn't like the phone to ring. It was hard to know whether it was correct to extrapolate that he didn't like Amy on the phone. Jill explained that her brothers emailed or texted their sister, but the correspondences had become business-like and curt. The spontaneity of a phone call or the prescient sharing of a story was gone. Jill feared that the siblings would drift apart if barriers to communications were set up. She expressed similar fears about Amy's loss of friendships. It was appearing to Jill that Amy was becoming more isolated and was losing contact with friends and family with whom she had previously been close. I couldn't help but remember the pretty, blonde girl whose phone "ribbited" in her bag during office visits. Where did that social girl go? I was mindful not to editorialize when Jill was expressing her concerns. She went on to tell me that she and two of her sons have gently expressed concerns to Amy about the relationship and more importantly, about her emerging isolation. Amy reassured them that she was happy and that planning the wedding was stressful, impressing upon them that whatever tension they perceived was certainly attributable to the pre-wedding preparations.

I gave Jill her anti-anxiety drug prescription and a few business cards for counselors in the area who may be able to help her sort out some feelings. I wished her well and reminded her that Amy was almost thirty years old and was adult enough to make her own decisions. It was a nauseatingly P.C. wrap up response on my part. I couldn't help but think that Amy was a girl with a lot of potential who may have missed a few developmental milestones along the way. A girl who may have some guilt about leaving her maternal home as she unwittingly served as surrogate spouse to her mother for years. A girl who may be about to sell herself short in choosing a mate as she approached the witching age of thirty years and wanted to start to think of having a family of her own. Or was Amy fine and in a very healthy and happy relationship? Was it refreshing that in this age of boundless communications, she and her future husband relished their quiet time? And was her mom being overly concerned, as life transitions can bring out worry in all of us?

On the way out of the office that day, Jill said that she'd need the prescription for the upcoming weekend. The two families would be getting together to look at tuxedos and discuss some wedding plans. Innocently enough, I asked where they would be shopping for the Tuxedos. Jill turned around, prescription in hand, and with a knowing lift of one eyebrow said, "Big and Tall."

***

I cannot begin to enumerate the number of stories I hear about how marriage alters irreparably the dynamics of a family or a social group. This story stands out for me as a particularly stark example of how one's marital choice can change the fabric of one's life and have relationship effects that ripple across generations. There are countless stories of mothers who no longer talk to their sons because of some dynamic with their daughters in-law or grandfathers who have to make appointments to see their new grandchildren due to some house-rule established by the new family. Relationships are complicated, and of course there are two—if not more—sides to every dynamic, but for me the take-home message is the same: Be careful who you marry.

It seems that our approach to finding a partner may be skewed. Dating services or friends often want you to itemize five traits you'd like to have in a spouse. This concept alone seems to oversimplify the process to the point of distortion. You feel like asking, "Do you want fries with that?" Who dubbed you judge and jury of another while staring at a computer screen with feet raised in furry slippers wearing a lush smoking jacket, pointing, clicking, and assessing the character of another person? I will argue that it is quite a bit easier to critique a prospective partner than it is to turn the scrutiny inward.

I would advise young people—or more mature people, for that matter—to know themselves, their goals, and their dreams before trying to unite with another. It seems that the single person should be able to answer at least a few basic questions first before he/she can look for a partner.

"How do *you* want to contribute to the world?"

"Where do *you* want to do it?"

I never asked Amy either of these questions and I am not a trained therapist, but I can't help but think that she wouldn't have had answers. She seemed to plug in a few criteria: tall, college graduate, add water, mix, and presto—insta-spouse! She was approaching thirty years old and her biological clock was ticking. What if long before thirty years old, she turned her attentions inward? What if she had the strength to demand an identity not defined by her relationship to her mother? What if she fearlessly dated, broke up, and recovered in a timeline keeping pace with her peers?

Of course, compromise is an integral part of every dynamic and relationship and, as a result, it would seem that this "wish list" paradigm for spouse acquisition may be questionable. An early, life-long investment in one's self is inarguably a good one. Then, no matter on which side of the fifty percent divorce statistic you fall, you'll always land on solid ground.

Chapter Four

THE HEADSHOT

In my grade school recollection
She had it all: smarts and good health
Her mom in full-length fur
Her dad exuded confidence and wealth.

Sitting in the classroom
Erect of posture she sat tall
Elbow straightened, hand raised proud
She was ready for it all.

Glasses with red rims
Magnified her baby blues
It seemed as if her life
Would be the one that you would choose.

There always was a party
Her mom—a gracious host
Hers were the birthdays every year
You looked forward to the most.

Like a curtain on a stage
Auburn curls they flanked her face
Flighty in her thoughts
Always a dream she'd want to chase.

She'd say, "I want to be an actress"
My name all lit up bright
I was named for royalty
It was meant to be in lights.

I guess a father's Santa hugs
A mother's doting song
Does not replace the love of peers
The feeling she belonged.

Behind the chauffeur and the limo
The tinted windows and the rims
Was a lost and lonely girl inside
Blocked vision out as well as in.

High on life was not a high enough
There was a dark and hollow space
Nothing could curtail the hurt
An aching, bleeding place.

Exsanguinating from her loss
Her sense of self was pale
She looked to others to restore the blush
Fluff up her ego which was frail.

Our self-concept—it's a portrait
From the brushstrokes of our peers
A stable loving family

Cannot buffer all the jeers.
Sometimes it's misperception
And no one's being mean
But it matters how you take the taunts
That's what you really glean.

The final party hosted
This one she couldn't make
Her gracious parents greeted guests
At her memorial—her wake.

Her headshot—it was beautiful
You couldn't help but think
What direction could her life have gone
If she never took a drink.

***

My doctor-patient relationships have shaped more than just my professional career. Coveted lessons and shared experiences have colored my outlook on life, shaped my goals as a parent, and altered my approach to friendships.

But doctors are people, too. Our personal experiences tint our professional outlook as well. My approach to patients and their families struggling with alcohol and drug addiction has been unapologetically altered by the personal loss of a dear friend. I hope that by sharing her story, I honor her memory, celebrate childhood friendship, and pledge to be the best doctor I can be for patients and families struggling with addiction and loss.

***

Donna was in the highest reading group in first grade. She read fluently and with perfect inflection. She'd occasionally adjust the bridge of her red-rimmed glasses as they inched down her sloped nose. Even that gesture exuded a certain confidence and made her appear the consummate intellectual (as much of an intellectual as you can appear in the first grade). I remember finding her glasses intriguing—a bit of a curiosity because few people required vision correction in the first grade class. Even fewer still required her thick, magnifying lenses, which enlarged her eyes to an unrealistic size, like two blue pools flanking her nose. Her mother always had her dressed in the finest fashions. I remember most notably her white stockings and her black Mary Janes. One could argue that this was the style then, but she always seemed to be dressed for an event that was happening right after school. There was no formal dress code and pants without holes or patches were allowed at school, but I don't recall her wearing pants often. A skirt or dress with white stockings and black maryjanes was her staple.

I also remember her posture. While other kids might slump in their chairs or fold in on themselves with a contortionist's flexibility—all four limbs off the floor, contained in the grade school chair-desk contraption—Donna wouldn't. She, by all accounts, was proper. Feet were crossed at the ankles, or her Mary Jane soles were at the ground and her rear end nestled deep in the seat so her spine aligned neatly with the chair back. She sat proper, erect, and ready. Looking back, some kids may have found her affected and snooty. I always found her interesting and sophisticated. It's all in the perception, I suppose.

To best know her, perhaps we should know her parents. Her dad, Steven, was by all accounts from a privileged beginning. Only the brightest boys of the finest breeding attended his boarding school. All dressed alike in their little lord Fauntleroy garb, the boys posed for their perfunctory class pictures which would grace the walls of the school marking the next class of up and rising stars. The alumni roster was a who's who of future doctors, lawyers, and businessmen. There was the expectation that the young graduates would go on to obtain advanced degrees and be pioneers in their respective fields. As young as ten years old, the boys were sent out of their family homes and off to their second "school family." As an only child, he relished the camaraderie and brotherhood of his dormitory life and was excited to play the role of perennially jovial young boy with the world at his fingertips.

Life back at home was a bit less lively for Steven. His father spent much of his day in his mahogany walled study and home office juggling various deals in different stages of development. Children were to be seen and not heard. As an only child, much of his play was with the house staff—cooks, maids, and cleaning crews. They especially enjoyed his breaks from school and his visits back home because he spiced up the house a bit and distracted them from his mother, who usually ruled the roost. His mother could predictably be found on the back porch in good weather and in the den in inclement weather with a book in hand and a martini within reach on the end table.

"Mother (never mom) why don't you ever have a lemonade or a tea like the other mothers?"

"First, Steven, because I am not like the other mothers. And second, because Nellie makes such a fine dry martini, it would be criminal to not ask for one."

All of this was said without averting her eyes from her reading. She suggested he go play and her long fingers curled around the stem of the martini glass as she "hmphed" to herself in response to something she'd read. Dismissed, but not dampened in spirit, he'd amble into the kitchen to see what Nellie and the others were up to.

Nellie and her brother Samuel both worked on the estate— she in the kitchen and he largely on the grounds. Nellie sang softly to herself as she fixed Samuel a sandwich, and he interjected the baritone chorus when appropriate. Beads of sweat traced his upper lip and perspiration stained his collar and armpits.

"Well hello Mr. Adams. It's hotter than blazes outside." Steven was referred to by the staff as "Mr." no matter that he was eleven years old.

"I haven't been out yet. Mother says I'm supposed to go play."

"Well there's no play in here. What are your plans?"

Ignoring the question, he asked, "What were you singing when I came in?"

"Oh, you liked that? Me and Nellie were singing a hymn from church."

"I didn't say I liked it. I just asked what you were singing," the boy smirked, delighted by his own smart remark.

"You're a quick one, there Mr. Adams" Samuel acknowledged holding up a finger as if to gesture *the first round goes to you.*

Steven couldn't help but notice Samuel's wide, callused palm and his darkened fingernails. Samuel was a very clean man and the boy knew that he'd just washed his hands if he was sitting down to lunch. Some stains are hard to wash off, he thought to himself.

"What goes on in your church?" Steven asked.

"A little sermon, a little singing, a little praying," Samuel answered in between sandwich bites.

"Do you like going?" he asked, almost timidly.

"Hmmm," Samuel pondered as he wiped his hand on a napkin. "Yeah, I suppose I like going. It keeps me grateful, keeps me singing too, I guess," Samuel answered.

"Mother says that church-going is not for us," Steven remarked. The words hung heavy in the kitchen and Nellie shot Samuel a look, summoning him to silence.

"Why don't you go change. I was just about to hose down the deck and if you're not careful, I might just get you wet by accident," Samuel interjected casually as he brought his lunch plates to the sink where Nellie extended her hand to receive them and smiled with a nod of approval.

And that was Donna's dad. Privileged, well schooled, and somewhat left to raise himself—buoyed forward by precocious questions and guided by open-ended answers.

Her mom's background was distinctly different. Raised along with her siblings by her capable grandmother, Agnes enjoyed a quiet life in the Southwest filled with old-fashioned values and spiritual guidance gotten through weekly church attendance. A naturally pretty girl, she was well received at school by teachers and fellow students alike. Her only socially awkward moments were when she was asked about her home life, or more specifically, her mother.

"Why do you live with your grandmother?" kids would ask. This was probably all innocent enough playground banter, but for her, this subject was sticky and one she didn't want to touch.

"My grandmother's around more so we figured it would be best."

"Where's your mom at then?"

"She's at auditions. She's very talented, you know. She may hit it big one day. Anyway, these fancy shows she's in—they're not performed here in this small town. They're in big cities with lights and bustling streets. She has to go where the work is, you know."

That type of response was usually satisfactory for the playground kids. The young girl was well liked and no one was going out of their way to find a soft spot to poke at. There was probably a cringe or two inside when she acknowledged to herself that this answer was only a half-truth. Her mother did have aspirations of being a performer and if Agnes resembled her at all, her mom may have been blessed with leading lady good looks, but the truth was that her mother was never too far from home. She lived in a single-wide trailer just on the outskirts of town and performed in a piano bar from time to time, but spent most of her days asleep and her nights awake drinking cheap wine out of a plastic cup. The altered and somewhat embellished version of the story went down a lot smoother and, if Agnes told that version often enough, she'd even come to believe it herself. Back then I don't know if they had formal court documents declaring guardianship or defining custody, but no such legalities seemed necessary in this case. Her mother relinquished her role as parent to her own mother and exchanged her children for a dream and a bottle.

Weekly church excursions with her grandmother were not only mandatory, but were also social outings. Christian values and faith united families in this small town, providing solid, common ground for friendships. Church socials were a safe way to meet and mingle with the other boys and girls of the town. Even-tempered and approachable, Agnes often enjoyed a full dance card. She was as excited as any young girl to go to these socials, but she didn't see them as the "husband prospecting" opportunity that so many of her friends did. She loved her small town and the wholesome values of her local church, but she couldn't help but wonder what else was out there. While singing her church solos, as her operatic soprano notes were sailing above the heads of the congregation, she couldn't help but wonder where else her voice could carry her.

That is a snapshot of Donna's parents' early childhood as seen through the lens of my own childhood friendship and as invariably tweaked by the compassionate allowances of memory. Steven went on to prestigious schools, attending a college and graduate school reflective of his family's expectations. He was a larger-than-life fellow, both in stature and in spirit. His appetite for adventure was at once his greatest strength and his greatest weakness. He bored easily and thrived on new projects and new ideas. His enthusiasm for life and learning was infectious and he was always on the verge of the "next big deal." Agnes, on the other hand, was practical and, although hopeful, was grounded enough to stay close to the confines of social roles. She earned a secretarial degree and pursued voice lessons. With formal instruction in voice, she became recognized as quite a talent in her small town and was determined to cultivate her gift while she honed her skills. It was a secretarial job in Chicago as well as the opportunity to sing outside of a church choir that took the small-town girl into the big city.

Agnes entered the secretarial pool in her pressed business skirt (a "congratulations on your first job" gift from her grandmother) and her dictation pad. She was informed at orientation earlier that day that she'd be working for a fairly new executive. She was told that he was quite an upstart and that he generally delegated many tasks to his assistants because he often worked on multiple projects at the same time. She assured the secretarial pool supervisor that she was up for the challenge and that she prided herself on her ability to multitask.

A burly man barreled through the double doors leading with his belly as his hands were full of files so precariously arranged that the papers were at risk of a shuffled, confetti fall to the floor. She hastened up from her chair and offered to straighten out the papers, taking the initiative to unload the files one at a time in an effort to support and assist her new executive. And so it happened. Steven, the bombastic adventurous, spirited dreamer married Agnes, the lovely, talented, church-going singer.

This curious union, born of chance and founded on love and mutual admiration, was the core of Donna's family. Her parents were singularly devoted to her and were openly prideful of any accomplishment, no matter how small. Given this, you may ask why was she plagued by weak coping skills and made brittle by fragile self-esteem? If these questions had answers, maybe everything would have ended differently.

I remember an incident in class involving graham crackers

and milk. The teacher would leave the room daily to fetch the snack and we were to sit quietly awaiting her return. The sitting around quietly concept was lost on some of my classmates and a room without teacher supervision seemed ripe for mischief. A boy named Alan thought that turning the lights off upon the teacher's exit and on when he heard the clippidy clop of her shoes approaching was genius. More than one student vociferously protested Alan's daily prank. I, for one, was too busy welling up with tears to protest too much and was made nervous by the lack of order. Finally, in a crescendo of panic, I began sobbing. There was one light flicker too many and the disobedience of rules broke me (I've always been a bit of a goody two shoes). Donna, the girl with the red-rimmed glasses, wriggled out of her desk-chair contraption with conviction and an exaggerated stomp. She huffed over to the light switch, flicked it on, and in a projected voice admonished Alan to leave the lights on and to not touch the switch again. This was met with a heavy silence, which paved the path for flung insults. Like darts at balloons, he shot back with name-calling: four eyes, blubber, bossy jerk . . .

I'm certain there were lots of times that I was called a baby because of my sniffling and crying, but I never remember that fazing me. I felt that I was justified to be upset by the lack of order and the disregard for the teacher's rules. I was frightened and powerless, which led me to tears of frustration. Even then, I didn't care who called me a baby because my feelings were authentic (albeit somewhat unrestrained). I'm being truthful when I say I don't remember being affected in the least by any name-calling. But what I *do* remember is watching the bravado knocked right out of my classmate as she stood vulnerable and alone at the light switch. She retaliated with a snide insult and sulked her way back to her desk. She was out like a lion and in like a lamb. The theatrics and affectation did not shield her well from jeers. It was as if she wore her skin inside out—nerve endings exposed and unprotected by an outer covering. I went on to become snack monitor, leaving the teacher behind to mind the classroom each day as I went off to the kitchen to get everyone's graham crackers and milk. My classmates waited behind with lights on and order restored. After the graham cracker and milk incident, I knew that I might have a friend in that girl. We may not have handled ourselves similarly in certain social settings, and she may have been more of an upstart than I in a classroom, but I knew she was loyal and she was true. What more could anyone ever ask of a friend?

We never shared a classroom again. My family moved and I changed school systems. Her gregarious and social parents kept our friendship intact in the early years with well-timed and engaging invitations. Were it not for her family's generosity of spirit, our bond would have likely fizzled, but it didn't. Birthday parties, New Year's Eve celebrations, proms, and graduations marked the milestones of our friendship.

I remember a particularly grand party when we were in middle school. I suppose that we were thirteen or fourteen years old. The party was at Donna's home; a three story, colonial-style monstrosity perched on a hill. There was valet parking arranged that night as only certain of the residential streets permitted cars and the guest list was long enough that vehicles would undoubtedly spill out of the circular driveway. Her father greeted men, women, and children alike with a bone-crushing hug. I say this somewhat seriously as he was reported to have fractured a petite woman's rib with his enthusiastic squeeze. I was always on the shorter side and felt particularly in danger of suffocation as my face aligned well with his protuberant belly. I had prepared a skillfully timed inhalation and came out of the hug unscathed if not a bit ruffled up. Coats were taken and whisked off to a predetermined location and her mother drifted in and out of rooms making introductions and answering questions about the furnishings. I remember feeling like a Lilliputian in the place. The ceilings were high, the rooms oversized, and the plush furnishings made large and custom to fit.

I was always made to feel like a relation and after a few introductions, was instructed by Donna to jump in the elevator to go to the third floor. This was her dad's home office and a place we could stay for the evening. The elevator had been installed because Donna's great grandmother was ailing and living with them. The stairs were too much for her, so the white-latticed elevator with the indwelling red velvet chair was installed for her. Agnes would say, "She took care of me when I was a girl. Now I can take care of her."

Up in the study, sucked into overstuffed, corduroy-upholstered chairs, we sat with legs dangling and stereo remote in hand. We caught up on the goings on in each of our schools. I loved my school. I had nice friends and was motivated to do well. I enjoyed every minute from bus ride there to bus ride home each day. I was surprised when Donna shared a different experience with me. She told me that she hated school and thought that many of her female classmates were snotty bitches. She wasn't all that interested in the subjects and would frequently not hand in an assignment because it looked like it was going to require extra efforts to complete.

I was shocked. Remember, I am the same kid who started crying when there was a little ruckus in a dimly lit classroom. I looked at my friend in disbelief who stared back at me with her deep, blue eyes. She had shed the glasses by then and was adept at the insertion of contact lenses, which I find disconcerting even now thinking back on it.

"What do you mean?" I asked.

"What do you mean what do I mean? The girls are bitches. The boys are jerks. And I don't see how any of these classes will help me when I'm an actress. I want to be on the stage. I don't want to be sitting in a classroom learning the Latin root for 'memory.' And I certainly don't want to plug numbers into algebraic equations. I could care less. Let's watch a DVD. My dad's just set up this high tech projector thing and I'm sure I can figure it out."

While assuring me repeatedly that yes, we were allowed to watch a DVD, and yes, her dad wouldn't mind if she touched his equipment, she fumbled through the DVD stack. Intrigued by gizmos and gadgets, Steven always had the latest computer, the most high tech phone, and the snazziest techno toys. I laughed when the screen descended from the ceiling as I thought of my house. We always had one TV in our home planted in the middle of the family room. Everyone had to watch the same program at the same time. Music and the buzz of muffled conversations floated up from three stories down where the adults were.

Opening a cabinet under the sound system, she held up a bottle by its neck and asked,

"Want a drink with your movie?"

"What is that?"

"Vodka. Grey Goose. Want any?"

"You better put that back. I'm sure your father has it for clients and stuff."

"Oh, he does. They probably toast deals with it. Want some?" she asked with chin tucked down and big eyes rolled up. I couldn't tell if she was being serious or not and concluded that she wasn't. She paused a little too long with Grey Goose in one hand and the color-adapted version of the Wizard of Oz in the other.

"No thanks," I said. And she placed the vodka back, put the DVD in, and settled into the overstuffed chair with the remote control.

The evening was great fun as were all of the events hosted by her parents. They graciously thanked each guest for coming and said that it wouldn't be long 'til the next get-together.

Donna had a birthday party every summer. Each one was spectacular and I, for one, looked forward to going. As time passed though, I began to notice that many of the kids on the guest list were children of her parents' friends. I never attended school with her except that one early elementary year and I expected to meet some classmates of hers at these parties. Instead, I'd recognize kids who'd attended various events at the home when they were accompanied by their parents. I never thought anything of this at the time. I was always seated in a position of honor next to the birthday girl and if you put a slice of custom-made, Disney character cake in front of me, preferably with blue, inorganic icing, I was happy!

Time passed, events came and went, and we grew up together, but separately. We graduated from high school the same year— me on an academic college track and her barely squeaking by as she freely admitted plans to enter a performing arts secondary school. She was always well spoken with a fine vocabulary. We spent a lot of time on the phone and so many conversations had passed between us. (Those were the days before texting and emails.) It baffled me how someone so naturally bright was barely squeaking by. I chalked it up to a lack of personal application and effort and never gave it much thought. She used to say that we were like the pair of friends in the movie *Beaches*. She was like Bette Midler- free-spirited, flighty, and talented and I was like the grounded, brunette woman in the movie, just without the daughter or the terminal disease.

She would croon, "You are the wind beneath my wings." and I would eye-roll, smile, and shake my head silently saying, "You're crazy."

Over the next ten years, lots of school happened for me and lots of life happened for her. Donna ultimately completed two out of the four years of her program and began auditioning. I'd hear about the odd audition here and there and there were countless jobs. I really mean countless, like too many to enumerate. Some lasted as little as six weeks: waitressing, hostessing, babysitting, retail, car sales . . . you name it, she did it.

"Don't you want to stay in one place so that you can get a set schedule and focus on auditions?" I asked.

"Listen, I do, but I couldn't possibly have stayed in my last job. Between the banal people working there and the menial tasks being asked of me, I had to leave."

"Yeah, but stocking shelves is part of retail. I know that sales is hard, but you're so good at it. Think of it as acting. It's like an audition with a guaranteed paycheck. Maybe you should just stick it out in one of these positions. A manager or supervisor might recognize your potential and promote you or something."

"Don't worry, hon. I've got a job interview next week with an up and coming company. I met the owner when I was selling men's suits last spring. We hit it off, and I think that's going to work out well."

"Ok, good luck. Keep me posted."

"Yep, I will. Luv ya." she chuckled because she knew that I'd answer, "Yep. Me too." She was much more expressive than I, and she'd back me into a gushy reciprocation whenever she could.

She'd always been a fuller figured girl, a little "hippy" by her own admission. Her weight began to oscillate wildly. I recall commenting that yoyo weight loss and weight gain was more stressful on the body than even suboptimal weight maintenance. I attributed this weight fluctuation to her changing lifestyle and to her late night jobs in food service. She must have had wardrobes in three different sizes. Again, I figured this was possible given the employee discounts offered to some retail sales associates and I assumed that when she got thin, it was because she hunkered down and began a fitness program. She dated some and I'd hear about work acquaintances here or there, but no names ever carried over from one job to the next.

It was a "love the one you're with" mentality of existing. Donna would always tell me that I was one of her best and loyal friends of which she had two. The other also was a young woman from elementary school, but college and a career had taken her out of the area, so their friendship subsisted largely of phone calls.

"You're not thinking of moving, right?" she'd ask.

"No. I want to do my training in the city if I can, so I hope to stay around here."

"Good. I'd miss you if you left."

"Well, I won't be leaving," I reassured.

"Good. 'Cause I luv yah, hon."

"Me too," I answered.

I don't know when the spiral started. I began to notice little things. We'd go out to dinner. I'd order a diet Coke and she'd order a bottle of wine. We finished the meal and the waiter capped off her glass, taking away the empty bottle.

"Isn't that a lot of wine for one person? Did you just finish the bottle?" I inquired. Not being a drinker, I always doubted my awareness of what was ordinary consumption.

"No, it really isn't. That kind is really light anyway. I feel fine," Donna answered confidently and not at all defensively. I was usually the driver so if she seemed fine, she was fine. My friend, the actress, starred in a role of her own creation every day. She just played the part so well that I never knew I was an audience member. Isn't that what actors do? They help you suspend disbelief enough for you to engage. They help you believe what you want to believe.

I was busy with an all-consuming medical training program and she was busy bouncing from job to job. There were gaps in our get-togethers that spanned months, but when we did reconnect, it was as if we never were apart. There was an occasion when we were in a car together. I was driving and we were headed to a Christmas party. The host was a friend of mine from high school and the guest attendance policy was "the more the merrier," so I brought Donna. Her cell phone rang and when she went to get it, she inadvertently hit "speaker." For a second, a strange man's voice was heard. He had an accent and was about to launch into a tirade about where something could be found when she hastily pressed the "silent" button. She listened for a second, shrugged, and said, "Wrong number."

"Who was that?" I asked, pretending not to have heard her.

"Wrong number. My cell number must be similar to someone else's. I've told them before but they keep dialing it anyway," she said with a sniffle and changed the subject. "Who's going to be at the party?" She popped open the visor mirror to have a last look at her face before we pulled into the apartment complex visitor parking lot. I wanted to enjoy our evening together and I didn't press her further on the matter.

Years later, it was 1:30 a.m. and my phone rang.

"Hon. It's me." she slurred. "Are you there?"

"Yes, I'm here. What's up? Are you ok?" I was sitting up in bed at this point somewhat annoyed that she'd call me all liquored up. "Are you drunk?" I accused.

"No, they have me all drugged up. It's hard to think?"

"Where are you? Who has you all drugged up?" I asked worried and thinking now she may be calling from an unmarked white van or something holed up at the side of the road.

"The doctors. I'm in the hospital. Oh which one am I at? I don't know. Is it morphine? I'm so itchy. My head's fuzzy," she rambled.

"You're in the hospital?!" I asked with growing alarm. "For what? What's wrong? Why are you in the hospital? Now focus! Tell me!" I shouted.

"I'm in the hospital. I needed to call you. They say that I have six weeks to live. I needed to call you." she said and started to drift off.

"Six weeks to live?! What are you talking about? What's wrong?" I asked in disbelief. "Now, stay awake. Tell me! What's wrong?"

"Too much hard living. I have six weeks to live." This she said with mustered clarity.

"This can't be true. What do you mean?" I pleaded.

"Hon, I can't talk more now. It's so late and I know you're an early riser. I needed to tell you though. I'm glad I remembered your number. We'll talk soon. I love ya, hon," and the line went dead.

"Me too," I said to myself, hanging up the receiver in disbelief. I checked the caller-ID on the phone, still hoping that she was in a drunken stupor and calling from home with another wild tale. I was frightened to see a hospital abbreviation on the phone and a call back number resembling a hospital operator telephone line.

The next day, I phoned her mother and confirmed that my worst fears were true. My friend's condition was terminal and indeed the doctors had forecasted that she would live another six weeks. Cirrhosis of the liver and subsequent organ failure would take her quickly. She'd likely not suffer, as natural toxins would build up, serving to auto-anesthetize her. She would drift in and out of a brain fog and then she would leave us.

Once Donna was released from the hospital into the care of her mother, I planned a visit. I went bearing lunch and a photo album I'd assembled of our shared memories from elementary school to adulthood. There were far too many clear plastic sheets at the end of the book that would never be filled with accompanying pictures. The door was ajar and her mother shouted to come in. Agnes was in the back, helping my friend to the bathroom. I entered and on the grand piano displayed facing the entryway was an eight-by-ten inch headshot of Donna. I couldn't help but think right then that I'd see this photograph again soon when we went to pay our respects. Blinking and shaking my head to erase the thought, I started to put out the lunch. Her mom came out at the same time apologizing for not having the place settings ready.

"She should be out in a minute. She's moving around more slowly these days," her mother explained.

I looked up to see Donna shuffling laboriously toward the table. Her legs had become heavy with extra fluid that her liver couldn't process and her kidneys couldn't expel. A dialysis catheter jutted out from her swollen neck and her face was distorted and bloated by disease. Dim lighting somewhat camouflaged her jaundice, but a sickly, yellow hue now coated her once-porcelain skin. Her big blue eyes and her tight curls were the only features recognizably hers. In fact, she wasn't wearing her contacts, but instead her glasses (she'd lost the red rims by this point, but still required significant magnification). After lunch, I walked her back to her room, draped towels over her bed and helped her raise her weeping legs. When she wasn't drifting off, we looked at the album together, reminiscing about our first grade class, our proms, my wedding, etc. I held the album and Donna pointed to the pictures and editorialized what she could.

"Will you look at my fat ass in that photo?! Whoever took that one should be shot," she'd assert. Or "You look great here. You've always been photogenic. Bitch!" And we'd laugh.

"Hon?"

"Yes?"

"You'll come to my service won't you?"

"What?"

"You're coming to my memorial service, right? Bring your folks. I'm afraid that no one will be there."

"I'll be there," I reassured. "Don't talk about that."

"I have to. It's going to happen. I know it. And I just don't want the place to be empty. You have to come."

Speechless, I held her hand and thought to myself how weak her grasp was in return.

"Of course I will be there," I answered trying not to let my voice shake.

"I have no friends, you know."

"You have me."

"I'm getting tired. I think I need to rest. I love you, my friend."

"I love you, too," I answered and I squeezed her hand for the last time.

Her memorial service was beautiful. Her father greeted guests with strong handshakes and big hugs in the lobby of the church. When I arrived and we met each other's eyes, no words were exchanged. Our embrace was so long it held up the line of entering visitors. Neither one of us wanted to release—clinging to one another before we had to say our final goodbyes to his beloved daughter and my beloved friend. Her mother sang at the service. We all marveled at her composure during the song. She later told us she was channeling her voice teacher from her childhood and had said a prayer that she'd get through it. After the last soprano note chimed, she turned away from the microphone and left the podium. You could see her shoulders shake with the pain of her muffled sobs. All of the choir ladies baked an item and we sat at round tables after the service. Agnes, the perpetual hostess, remarked on the nice turn-out and the tasty homemade desserts. Family friends, choir members, and relatives gathered that night to pay their respects. Looking back, I hope that she knew that her last wish was granted. The place wasn't empty.

***

Throughout my career, I've seen young people fall victim to drug and alcohol abuse. I've tried to find a common theme, something that links the encounters, threading them neatly like strung popcorn. No such unifying factor exists, but I will say that inappropriate coping seems to play a role in almost all drug and alcohol abuse stories. As soon as someone begins to self-medicate with alcohol, the problem has begun. I will assert that the sales rep in a high-pressure job who drinks a beer or two to "wind down" after work should be concerned. The college student who sees graduation approaching and is no closer to knowing what he wants to be when he grows up and binge-drinks the weekends away to forget should be concerned. And, the young girl who seemingly has everything except the easy acceptance of her peers who drinks to numb her pain should be concerned. It's hard to hone coping skills to manage mounting pressures. It's hard to introspect and access the real answer to the question: "What do I want to do? What makes me tick?" And it's hard to self-reflect and ask: "Why is fitting in hard for me, and what can I do to change that?"

There's a lot of hard work we do in life but there is no greater toil than sculpting, knowing, and accepting ourselves. My friend tried to cheat hard work and self-application in more than one venue, but her terminal error was deciding to self-medicate her social sorrows with alcohol. I can't help but wonder if she'd had the tenacity and interest to explore the mounting problem of her social acceptance (or lack thereof), would the story have ended differently? I can't even say for certain that she ever really had any horrible experiences in school socially. After all, we didn't attend the same school except for one elementary classroom year. But in this case as in many, perception is reality. And if she thought she did, she did. Instead of navigating the scenes, she chose to dilute her discomfort, a choice made more dangerous by her genetic predisposition to overuse alcohol. If I had to impart any advice, I'd quote the cliché, "You can run, but you can't hide." A chemical escape may seem tempting, but it marks only a brief curtain close. The second act always picks up where the first left off. I watched as not a single of my friend's hopes were realized. There was no marriage, no children, no bright lights, no acting, no applause. I'd like to hope that I've grown wiser, ebbing and flowing with my patients on their journeys through addiction and recovery. I've learned through countless patient encounters that the strongest, most resilient people seem to have a sense of ownership over their own lives. They seem to be empowered by the belief that not even bad times in their life are worth erasing.

Even on Donna's deathbed, she was concerned about her acceptance. Breaking through her cirrhotic haze was the fear that her memorial service wouldn't be well attended. It would seem that the very vulnerability she tried to drown in drink haunted her even in her foggy, encephalopathic sobriety.

To all of the parents who have struggled with their child's addiction and to all of the children who have struggled with their own sobriety, I applaud you. Denial is tempting, but regret is haunting and so relentless. Early intervention is everything when it comes to breaking the pattern of addiction. Looking back with compassionate allowances, I think that I saw signs of my friend's misuse of alcohol and her subsequent derailment. I don't feel guilty and neither should anyone who loved her. After all, you can't help people unless they're willing to help themselves. I once quoted this phrase to a dad struggling with his son's addiction. I was trying to relieve him of some burden of responsibility.

Ironically, he said,

"Yeah, I hear you, but you know what that is? That's a cop-out. It always comes back to the parent. You can say that. The psychiatrist can say that. And the IOP (intensive outpatient) drug and alcohol program can say that. But I can't. He's my son and I won't stop until he's sober. I won't stop until he knows he's worth something. I'm going to run now. It's 'family night' at the IOP and I want us to be there on time. Thanks for everything, doc."

"No problem. Good Luck."

Chapter Five

THE LOST BOY

When you look into a newborn's face
Swaddled tight against your chest
Optimistic, hopeful
Prepared to offer him the best

Your breathing starts to slow
Your anxiety abates
The hope of life unmarred
His future, a blank slate

His simple wants, his simple needs
Each one, yours to satisfy
Ticking off the tasks at hand
Those early years fly by

Something changed along the way
It wasn't simple anymore
What you'd give to turn the clock back
Those baby memories restored

But life tics on regardless
A cruel and ruthless boss
Obstacles and sadness
Into a tangled web you're tossed

You wish that you could fix it
A shattered dream, a broken heart
You cannot live his life for him
Just because you gave its start

You must maintain your distance
Watch him fall and watch him flail
Guard against self-injury
Himself alone he must impale

Is your love enough to heal him?
No—of this you can be sure
Only love of self will help him
And this love, it must be pure

Watchful waiting is the only choice
Hold hope close and swaddle tight
He alone can mend his ways
And choose the cleaner fight

***

"Elaine?"

"Yes."

"It's Cheryl. We've called the ambulance. It's Bobby. At first he wasn't responsive, but the paramedics worked on him and they said he's breathing now."

"Thank goodness."

"Yes," she sighed. "Bob and I are following them to the ER."

"Ok. Good luck. I'll wait to hear from the ER doc and we'll be in touch."

"Ok. Thanks Elaine. We'll talk soon."

Her speech was pressured and her address familiar. It was not the first time that Cheryl had activated 911 for her son. We'd long since dispensed with the formality of Dr. and Mrs. It was Elaine and Cheryl.

I knew that it wouldn't be long before the ER called so I started getting dressed and ready to go in. Bobby would be triaged as top priority especially since he was being brought in by EMS. I wondered if this was like the last time. The family dog had found Bobby unresponsive in the weight room and began barking incessantly. An initially irritated and later frantic Cheryl had been lured into the weight room only to find Bobby face-down on the floor, his head inches away from a barbell. Back then, some narcan and a stern warning was all that EMS workers needed to give Bobby. This event already seemed more serious.

The ER knows no time. Incandescent lights fluoresce the halls twenty-four hours a day and emergency rooms always seem devoid of windows. The lights are artificial and the smell is a manufactured Clorox/ammonia blend doused to conceal the stench of vomit, bloody stool, or just general sickness. We no longer list patient names and locations on the wall for the purposes of privacy, so I, like most community docs, squint and strain through the ER gurneys looking for familiar colleagues or patients. That night was particularly packed and a random room sweep looking for Bobby seemed unproductive. I spotted an ER doc I knew and made my way over to him. One hand was on his cordless phone and the other on the computer mouse. With a spare finger and a nod, he communicated: "Hi, Elaine. Give me a minute and I'll fill you in on your young man . . . " The seat next to him was empty and it soon became clear why as I sank unceremoniously to the floor.

"We've been meaning to call maintenance. That chair's broken," he said shutting off the phone and looking down at me.

"Yes. It is," I acknowledged, my knees unnaturally bent.

"How's Bobby?"

Confused, he paused a moment to clarify. "Robert? Twenty-three-year-old overdose? He's in room four. He's groggy, but conscious. Breathing on his own. The paramedics got there in time," he continued. "In fact, I was just about to call Poison Control. We suspect a cocktail of drugs: fentanyl, Lexapro, and ink from a jet printer."

"Ink?!" I asked in disbelief—virtually reclined now as the spring on the back of the chair was evidently broken too.

"Are you comfortable down there?" he smirked.

"It's not about me. Seriously, ink?"

"The paramedics thought they saw remnants in his mouth when they did a finger sweep to check his airway. Nothing surprises me anymore. I'll call Poison. He's in four," he said, extending a hand to help me to my feet.

I approached room four cautiously as the curtain was drawn. I wasn't sure if this was for just discretionary reasons or if one of the nurses was back there with him. Peeking my head around the curtain corner, I saw Cheryl seated at the gurney-side chair and Big Bob standing and staring mindlessly at the telemetry box. I knew that he owned his own accounting firm and was unlikely to be familiar with all of the vital sign parameters of the bedside cardiac monitor. Arms folded with an unblinking stare, he paced. When I caught a glimpse of Bobby, it was clear why Big Bob would rather eye-avert feigning attention to the glowing lines of the heart rate and respiration tracings. If I didn't know that Bobby was alive, I would have sworn that he was dead. His cheeks were bloated with subtle periorbital swelling closing his eyes just enough for his lashes to graze against one another, but not enough for his eyes to fully shut. I made a mental note to tell the nurse about it so she could apply some natural tears or lubricant. We didn't need to add corneal abrasions to our growing list of problems. And his coloring was off. His skin was pasty and his limbs flaccid. His shirt had been cut off in the ER and some frayed gray T-shirt fragments stuck out from beneath his shoulders like jagged wings.

The eerie silence was broken by Cheryl looking up and saying,

"Elaine, thanks for coming. They think he'll be alright." Big Bob just turned around and bent down for a hug. He was the epitome of the strong, silent-type.

"Of course. If you're here, I'm here. I'm sorry about this," I said looking at Bobby's motionless body. "I've been briefed a bit by the ER doc already, but do you know what happened?"

Cheryl recounted the horror of finding Bobby unresponsive and calling 911. She watched as if in a third dimension as the EMS fellows wordlessly worked on what appeared to be Bobby's lifeless body. They didn't say much as they rhythmically loaded him onto a stretcher and, on the count of three, hoisted him into the ambulance among the clanging of folding wheels and the clap of the cool metal doors closing. They felt it best that the parents follow them to the hospital in a car, so she was unable to share any of the events of the ambulance ride.

Just then, the alarm started sounding, a piercing, relentless beeping. I looked up at the monitor and it seemed that the pulse oximeter wasn't registering. I fished under the hospital issue white linens to find that the device had slipped off Bobby's finger and reattaching it put a swift end to the noise. It hardly seemed right that he should continue to rest in his drug-filled haze while the three of us endured a moment of panic at the suggestion that he'd stopped breathing. I explained to his parents that he'd be going to a monitored bed on the neurology floor. Since his airway didn't seem compromised, an ICU bed wasn't necessary at this time, but we'd watch him closely. I also explained that because the circumstances of the overdose were unclear, I'd be contacting psychiatry and Bobby would have a one-to-one. They nodded in taciturn agreement. I made my way to the head of the stretcher, leaned over and tried to wake Bobby with my voice. When that was unsuccessful, I performed a sternal rub while saying that we would take good care of him and that I'd meet him upstairs. At the pressure of my knuckle digging into his sternum, he moaned and his eyes flickered. His parents seemed relieved at his responsiveness. I, too, was relieved, but I was also happy that I'd caused him enough discomfort to stimulate him. Somehow, it didn't seem right that he should rest so comfortably amongst such pain.

The next morning I found him sleeping with eyeshades on. They looked like the kind that used to come in a plastic wrap from the airlines back in the day when free gifts and snacks were given. The aide was curled up in a geri-chair next to the bed, the glow of her iPhone illuminating a triangle around her mouth and nose. I whispered, "good morning," to her and she looked up and waved. I gave his arm a gentle tap, then a firmer one.

"Hey. How are you?" I asked in a stage whisper. He stirred, peeking out from under his eye covering.

"Oh. Hey," he said, pushing himself up. Hospital beds have a habit of swallowing their inhabitants.

"What the hell happened?"

Pulling off his eyeshades with one hand and running his free hand through his hair, he said,

"It's complicated."

"Yes. Ink from a jet printer?"

"Yeah. That was stupid."

"I'd say that only scratches the surface of stupid. Seriously, do you feel ok?"

"I feel ok. I'm tired, but ok."

"We are all prepared to help you if you want help. But I can't want it more than you do."

"I know. I've got to get my act together."

"We'll help you do that, but you have to want it more than anyone else—more than Mom and Dad, more than me," I reiterated. "Let me tell you about the day's events. The psychiatrist will come by and I suggest that you take advantage of his expertise. You'll keep the cardiac monitor on for the next couple of days. If there are no arrhythmias or concerns, we'll probably be able to discontinue it and you can move around a little more freely as long as you don't mind company," I gestured over to the one-to-one who hadn't yet looked up from her phone.

"Ok. Thank you," he said, rubbing his eyes. Perhaps he thought he'd wake up somewhere else if he rubbed hard enough. "This is going to kill my parents."

"I think they've already died a couple of times and keep coming back. They're resilient. But I'm glad to hear that you're thinking of them and their feelings."

"Yea. I really screwed up."

"Yes. No argument here. Listen, you're a great guy with so much to offer, but *you* have to believe it. *You* have to believe you're worth more."

He nodded wordlessly.

"Ok, so you've got today's plan. Behave yourself and I'll see you tomorrow. Remember, I'm an early bird, so I may interrupt your beauty sleep. I know you can afford it," I said cheekily.

He smiled and turned to the aide who was now politely listening to our conversation.

"What do you think? Quite a specimen? Huh," and he spiked up his thick almost black hair so it stood up at unnatural angles.

"Not bad," she smirked, and it was nice to hear her speak. The job of being a human shadow could be an awkward one at best, but Bobby would change that. I left the hospital room to him reaching for the television flipper asking what channel she'd like it on.

I sat in the fishbowl of computer terminals among the night shift workers finishing their documentation. Violent clicking and tapping filled the otherwise silent, dimly lit work station. I finished charting today's plan of care for Bobby and made a mental note that the grad student in my office would have to call the psychiatrist for an inpatient consult once his office opened. I was walking off the floor looking down at my patient list to strategize which stairwell would put me closest to my next stop when I saw a nurse poke her head out of a hospital room and shout out:

"Is anyone free to give a boost in room forty-four?!"

Another one swallowed by a hospital bed. It's like quicksand, I thought to myself turning the corner leaving the floor.

The day was filled with data accumulation, test acquisition, consults, and chart checking. We'd done this before, albeit this time seemed more grave. Ultimately, the psychiatrist felt that Bobby was competent to make his own decisions and a discharge plan to an inpatient drug and alcohol facility was recommended. I never did inquire whether the overdose was intentional or accidental and interestingly, there was no overt clarification of this in the psychiatrist's consult. I supposed that, in the end analysis, it didn't matter much.

The following morning, I walked into Bobby's room and he was holding court with a new one-to-one and his nurse at the head of his bed, necks craning to see a YouTube video on his phone. They were laughing animatedly and talking over one another in dynamic commentary.

"Am I invited?" I asked, entering without announcing myself. If I didn't so like being a doctor, I would have gotten a complex by now. A doctor entering that scene is like a principal entering a classroom. A gray hush overcomes the room and all of the sunny faces fade. "I didn't mean to interrupt."

"No, not at all," the nurse reassured politely. "I've got charting to do. Good luck, Bobby. The nurse coming on will be Charlotte. Show her the video if there's time. She will go crazy."

"Will do. Thanks Joan," he said, digging in the sheets for the buried phone charger. With phone plugged in and settled on the bedside end table, he looked up.

"Hey, doc."

"Hey," I said with a grand, queen's wave. "Bobby, it's d-day. What did you decide?"

"I'll go. The shrink gave me three inpatient rehabs around here. I think the case management lady is checking into insurance coverage."

"I'm glad and relieved to hear it. You know that this isn't a panacea. It's a three-to-seven day stay—a jump start. The real work starts when you get released."

"Yep. I know. I've got to get my act together."

"Ok then. I'm not going to say good luck because it's not a matter of luck. You're important enough to make this a priority. Without sobriety, you'll have nothing. No job. No social life. No future. I don't mean to sound preachy. I just want you to remember when you're getting discharged from wherever."

"I know. I've got it. Thanks for everything. Take care of mom and pops for me," he said, extending his hand.

Meeting his hand I said,

"I will. You're in my thoughts."

"Thanks, doc. Appreciate it."

I left the room not knowing whether to shake him or hug him. I would likely hear from Big Bob later that day regarding their choice of rehab. We'd never done an inpatient rehab before—just an IOP (intensive outpatient program). Walking down the empty hallway at that hour of the morning, I cursed my choice of shoes. The clap of my heels seemed annoyingly loud and if I tried to walk just on the ball of my feet, the shoes squeaked. I apologized to a loan custodian coming my way.

"I'm sorry. I'm very noisy today."

Amused, he smiled and said, "No crime in being noisy. Have a nice day doc."

"Thanks." I squeaked and clapped my way to the nearest stairwell.

I headed to the office after hospital rounds and entered the back way. I dropped my bag and plugged my phone in the shelving unit. Fortunately, the office hallway was carpeted so I was able to stealthily head up front to see if anyone was in yet. No one had arrived so I took this as an opportunity to look through the office candy jar and pilfer my preferred items. Stash in hand, I noticed the blinking message machine light.

"Hi everyone. It's Cheryl. Thanks for all you're doing to help us. When you get this message, can someone please have the doctor call me back? I wanted to go over a few discharge plan options we're considering. Thanks again for everything. Please use my cell number when you call back because I may be on my way to the hospital. Ok, then. Bye."

I liked the office before the day started. I usually did a quick sweep of things before folks arrived: lights on, magazines straightened, radio set to the country station . . . I balanced candies with my free hand, open like a tray for fear that they'd melt in a closed fist and with the other, I unlocked the door. It was persnickety and had a tendency to stick in humid weather. This way, I'd spare someone fumbling with a key to get in. I'd call Cheryl from the back office.

"Cheryl? Elaine Holt."

"Oh. Thanks for calling. I'm glad I didn't miss you. Cell reception in the hospital is terrible. I've just pulled in the parking lot. Let me get my ticket . . . " I could hear her fumbling to reach the ticket dispenser. "I'm sorry. One second," she strained. "I always park too far from these things." I could hear the car door open and close as she miscalculated her arm reach in relation to the parking ticket machine. "Ok. I'm settled now. Sorry about that."

"No problem. How are you holding up?"

"Oh. We're ok. Glad Bobby's ok, but we're getting tired. How's he doing?" she asked.

"Who? The Mayor? He's fine, somewhat alarmingly fine, I'd say."

"Uggh. Do you think he gets it?"

"In all honesty, I'm not sure. Thankfully, he's physically fine and there doesn't seem to be any lasting medical concern from the overdose. Does he 'get' it? I don't know."

"The psychiatrist advised an inpatient stay and the case management lady says that there are two places in the area that are covered under our insurance. What do you think?"

"I think that we have no choice. If experts are suggesting an inpatient stay, then that's what we have to pursue. But, like I told Bobby, this is not a cure all. The inpatient stay merely buys us a few days to generate plan B."

"Ok. I know and we figured that. I think that's Bob pulling in the lot now. We have some family meeting for discharge planning. I'm going to run. Thanks again and we'll keep you posted." And as she hung up the phone her voice trailed off, "Bob, over here . . . "

I rested my head on my high-back, plush office chair. I was probably appropriately neutral in tone with Cheryl, but in the silence of an empty office, I heard a different voice in my head. I wasn't optimistic. Bobby didn't seem scared enough to me. I didn't think that this was the nadir for him. If sucking on a printer cartridge and snorting fentanyl wasn't a low point, I didn't know what was. Just then, I heard the startling sound of the front door hitting the rubber stopper followed by a muffled expletive. I guessed that unbolting the door didn't resolve the sticking problem and made a mental note to look into that over the weekend. I headed up to the lobby to let the receptionist know that I was back from hospital rounds.

"Hi," I said. "What does today look like?" There was a time early in my career when I reviewed the schedule of appointments the night before, but no longer.

"Hold on. Let me pull the schedule up," she said readjusting her reading glasses and fumbling with the mouse. "How's Bobby anyway? This could take a minute to warm up." She motioned to the computer screen and sat back in her chair.

"Fine. Probably headed to rehab today so we'll see."

"They're such a nice family. I hope he does well."

"Yep. Jury's out. It's up to him now."

"Come around here so you can see this better. It could get pretty busy around 11 a.m., so watch the chitchat."

"I'm very good with time management," I assert indignantly.

"Yes. That's true in general, but there are a few folks here who could suck you in. Here, for instance, watch the 10:45, he talks a lot and very slowly," she warned, tapping the screen. "And what about the 10:30? She wouldn't say what she was coming in for so we weren't sure how much time to allot." Scrutinizing the schedule more closely, she added, "and the 11 o'clock may need the ramp."

I looked more closely, squinting a little. The bright lights of a computer screen have always bothered my eyes, but I've postponed a visit to the ophthalmologist for an embarrassingly long time.

"Really? I don't recall Barbara needing a ramp?"

"I don't know. Her husband called and said that she might need it. He said that it depends on the day. I asked him to let us know thirty minutes before he arrives so that we can have it set up for her."

"Ok. That's good. And I promise to pace myself," I smirked.

"You laugh, but I'm the one they stare at if you run more than fifteen minutes behind schedule. Our patients are used to punctuality, and there are only so many People magazines a person can flip through."

"Agreed. I won't let anyone wait. In fact, I see someone pulling in now. I'll head back and get myself organized."

"Good idea." She dismissed me, returning to the fax machine to sort the papers that came in overnight.

Many doctors do exclusively outpatient work now and have hospitalists manage their inpatients. I'm sure that the patients are well cared for and perhaps that model is more time efficient, but I still enjoyed the variety of seeing both inpatients and outpatients. I enjoyed starting the day (albeit early) with the quiet of the hospital followed by the crescendo of a somewhat condensed, office-based day. The morning commenced and progressed with its customary rhythm, each in her choreographed role. The front staffer performing check-in and check-out, the grad student on the phone in the back office, and the med tech processing blood specimens in the lab. I'd been a good steward of the time and managed to keep each appointment confined to its allotted slot without any hiccups or delays.

The receptionist came into the clinical area and announced, "I'm going to get the ramp. Listen for the door please." And she reached for the purple, latex-free exam gloves.

I handed some blood specimens to the lab tech at the same time that the grad student looked up and said, "Hospital nurse for you on line two." Snapping my pink gloves off, I washed my hands so I could take the call.

"Thanks," I shouted over running water and the whirr of the spinning centrifuge. "Hi."

"Dr. Holt?"

"Yes."

"It's Sonya from seven east. I'm taking care of Robert. They've decided to go to rehab. The parents are here and they're transporting him. I just need an order to discontinue the telemetry monitor so he can go."

"Oh. Of course. I should have done that when I was there earlier."

"That's ok. I'll take care of it."

"Before you go, how is everyone?"

"Fine."

"The parents? The kid? All seems fine."

"Yep. They're talking and laughing and just waiting for me to disconnect him so they can go."

"Hmmm. Ok," I paused, "of course discontinue the telemetry."

"Great. Thanks, Dr. Holt."

In the time I was on the phone, the wheelchair ramp had been set up and Barbara had already been placed in one of the exam rooms.

"Barbara, what's new and exciting?"

"Well this is new, but not exciting," she said, gesturing to the wheelchair. "And my liver lesions are new, but also not exciting."

"Your oncologist is particularly good at sending consult notes over. I was sorry to hear it."

"Yeah. I've been on borrowed time really for the last seven years, so I think it's all catching up to me."

"Are you uncomfortable?"

"No. I've got a pill for this and a lollypop for that and a whole bag of tricks for anything that ails me."

"I'm sure I can't help much, but what can I do?"

"Well, believe it or not, I'm here for a well visit. Ron gets a break on his premium if we all come for physical exams. I know that it seems ridiculous, but I'm here for my 'annual' visit," she said, putting finger quotes around "annual" and sighing with a resigned smile.

"What arm am I allowed to use?"

"The left only." She rolled up her sleeve, demonstrating her familiarity with the whole process. "I like the pink gloves. Matches your dress."

"Thanks a millie," I said, tying the tourniquet and lining all the blood tubes up on the end table while balancing a gauze and a Band-Aid on my knee.

"I think that the gal up front had purple."

"Yes. Purple is medium and pink is small. I vowed that if I ever had my own office, quick stick, I would use only cloth exam gowns and I would have any color gloves I wanted."

She guffawed, "You go girl."

"Ah, the little things," I said unsnapping the tourniquet, inverting the speckled tube several times. "Barb, do you think that you've wrapped up a lot of loose ends. Is there anything else or anyone else you need? I can't do much at this point, but do you need any help at home?"

"No. I think that we have everything pretty much covered. I can get around the house without the wheelchair. I just need to hear from my son, but you can't make that happen." I knew that Barbara and Ron had five children, two sons, three daughters. The eldest son, Ron had once said, "was off the deep end," but he'd never elaborated and I'd never pried.

"Is your son in the service?"

"No. He's a drug addict," she lamented. We did everything. At least I know that. *I did everything* in my power to help him. I raised four other high-functioning kids and I suppose that I'll never know what went wrong."

"I'm very sorry to hear that. You did nothing wrong. You couldn't have raised four other kids into adulthood if you were doing something wrong."

"I know that. I've been to Al-Anon meetings. I have no regrets. It's just that now I'm here," she gestured grandly around the exam room. "I'm at my last 'annual well visit'," she says again with mock quotations, "and the reality is . . . I may leave this earth and not be able to say goodbye to my firstborn son. None of the other kids stay in touch with him. They have their own families to protect and I get it. At least they have each other. They're all quite close. Ron and I haven't kept anything from them either. They know that the chemo is no longer working."

"There's nothing I can say to make this issue with your son better. I do remember you saying in the past that he's been out of touch."

"We hear from him every six months or so. To be honest with you, I am sorry to admit that I don't even know where he lives. I don't know if he's in a crack den somewhere or in a men's shelter? He's always had an open invitation to come home, but with the one condition that he'd want to clean up, and he's never wanted to."

"Maybe we can hope that he calls?"

"That's all I can do," she said, pausing for a moment. "How are things with you? Are your kids getting ready for school?"

"Let me just get this blood to the lab and I'll be right back to fill you in."

I couldn't help but think of Bobby during my brief walk to the lab. Would Cheryl and I one day have a similar conversation? Or, on the contrary, would she and Big Bob look back and shake their heads at the time Bobby had a near fatal overdose? Would they one day be able to share news of his great job, a wedding, and his adult life with a renewed sense of purpose? I put the lab specimens on the counter saying to no one in particular, "These are Barb's." Walking to the exam room I said, "Knock, knock," almost as a formality, already half opening the door.

"I'm where you left me."

"Ok. So where were we?" I said, sitting on my blue stool and shooting across the room making a mental note of what a good choice the no skid-tile was for the exam room floors.

The rest of Barbara's well visit was uneventful and we went through a cursory physical exam with some light banter. She gave me tips on where to find wigs locally and I spoke briefly of the kids' transition back to school. We ended the office visit with a hug, and I quickly flipped through a mental rolodex of salutations.

"Be well."

"See you next time."

"Have a good weekend." None seemed quite right and I settled on, "Please call me if you need anything. Have Ron do the same."

"Will do. In fact, you can send him in here to help maneuver the chair. It's a tight squeeze around corners."

Our avoidance of the topic sufficed as our goodbye. We both knew that it was likely she'd never have another office visit. I left the room and cued the lab tech to fetch Ron from the waiting room so they both could help Barbara out. Heading back to my office, I picked up my "RECEIVED" stamper and started to ink up the new items in my "UNIMPORTANT" pile. That pile was to be distinguished from my "IMPORTANT" and "VERY IMPORTANT" piles respectively. It was satisfying coming down hard with the stamper, marking each document "RECEIVED" and throwing the chart (at times too vigorously) into the fourth and final pile labeled "TO FILE." The noise of the stamper muffled the clanking and creaking of the wheelchair as it was rolled backwards down the metal slip and onto the ramp. Tucked away in the back office with my pile of documents, I couldn't see her leave.

It would be at least six months before I'd see Bobby again. The brief stay in the insurance-approved rehab had led to a thirty-day stay in a privately funded one. From there, he transitioned to what used to be called a halfway house, but now I think some call it a sober living community. And that marked his bridge back home. He was required to have a check-up with his regular medical doctor and, of course, his addiction specialist and then he'd be accepted into an IOP and transition back into life. The day before, we'd received a negative urine tox screen and some lab work over the fax in time for his appointment today. He was already in a room with vitals charted when I entered extending my hand asserting,

"Well, you look good on paper! We received your stats yesterday."

"Haha. Thanks." He was always quick-witted and plucky with a joke. "If you think that's good, let me show you what I have for an encore. It's an abdominal ultrasound. This was done a few months ago," he said, reaching to hand me the report. "I've dropped about twenty pounds since that was done,.."

"I was going to comment on how trim you look, but you beat me to it." Not looking up, I read off the report:

Diffusely increased echogenicity and coarsened echotexture consistent with fatty infiltration of the liver.

"Nice . . . a 'fatty liver,' " I said with mock appreciation for what seemed an uncomplimentary description. "In light of your weight loss, cleaner lifestyle, and now normalized liver function tests, we shouldn't have to worry too much about this. The liver is a forgiving organ, but you don't want to press your luck."

"Nope. I've got to stay on track. I've already met with the therapist, and once you clear me, I will start the IOP."

"Where will you go?"

"One out by my parents' place. They meet from 6 p.m. to 10 p.m. Monday through Thursday. This way, I can get some kind of a job. The P's say I need to cover some of my expenses if I'm going to be living at home."

"That's fair, right?"

"Absolutely," he quickly asserted without any reservation.

"I'm so glad to see you looking and feeling well."

"Thanks."

"What kind of work will you try to do?"

"Well, at this point, I'm not picky. I don't have any wheels right now."

I seemed to remember something about not driving for a while, but I didn't know the details. "Fair enough. Well, it's a good thing that there are a lot of public transportation options around here. You'll find something," I said reassuringly. We completed the exam and were wrapping up. The IOP physical form was brief and Bobby would be able to leave with it filled out. With my hand on the doorknob preparing to leave the exam room, I turned and said, "Bobby, let me take this form with me. I'll fill it out, make a copy and bring it up front for you. Can you wait in the lobby for a minute?"

"Sure. Jennifer dropped me off. She's at Starbucks now. She thinks it's great that my parents asked her to give me a ride here."

"Chauffeuring her big brother around . . . I'm sure she loves that."

"Yes, and I'm sure she'll never let me forget it," he said, rising from the chair and heading towards the lobby.

"Ok. It'll just be one minute. Catch up on your gossip out there. I have some new magazines."

"Yeah. Thanks. And . . . thanks for everything—the hospital stuff, helping my parents out," he said, blushing a bit. "I really appreciate it."

"No need for thanks, and I hope that I'm always here to help you out, but let's never have an instant replay of our last hospital stay, huh? Once was enough."

"Agreed. I'll wait up front." He walked toward the lobby fumbling with his phone, no doubt texting Jennifer that he was ready for pickup.

A few months later, a carefully clipped square from the local newspaper was laid deliberately in the middle of my desk where I'd see it. Any important news about local medical happenings, curious events from the police blotter, and, most important, obituaries found themselves in that spot as staffers were determined to keep me in the know. I picked up the clipping before I even put my bag down. It was Barbara's obituary. It said that she was the loving mother to five children and each were named in order of birth. Of course, it mentioned Ron and their forty-eight year union. It mentioned her charitable contributions and her career in teaching, but I kept coming back to her five children. I wondered if she'd ever heard from her son? If she did, was he in any condition to remember the call? Did he arrive at his mother's funeral? If he did, was he welcomed by his siblings? Or was their resentment too fresh, too raw from the suffering he'd caused? I'd never know, and I turned to throw the newspaper clipping in the garbage.

"Hey, is that you?" the receptionist shouted from the front. "I cut out Barbara's obituary for you."

"Yes. I just read it. Thanks," I shouted back, putting my bag down.

"Sad. She was a nice lady."

"Yep. She was." I reached for one of my condolence cards so I could send a note to Ron.

It's natural to wonder about the "Lost Boy," but perhaps what gnaws at us even more are the people he leaves in his wake. It was with noble strength that Barbara met the end of her illness and managed her unresolved heartache. How did she not perseverate and run sundry scenarios endlessly in her mind churning herself into a state of panic and unrest? Perhaps the debility of her illness stripped her of the energy required to be emotionally self-destructive? Or perhaps she was at peace. I'd like to believe that she was leaving this earth with the deep resolve that there were no regrets.

Similarly, I'd like to believe that Cheryl and Big Bob know what amazing people they are and additionally what amazing parents they are. I've always marveled at how parents of addicted kids can remain standing and continue functioning. How do they not fall under the weight of limitless worry or go crazy from cycling tragic endings in their minds? How do they not wake up in cold sweats questioning whether the phone call they received about their child's untimely death was real or dreamed? Maybe they do all of those things, but I will always be impressed by the public face these parents manage to wear.

I'd never know what happened at the end of Barbara's life. I'd see Ron and some of the daughters for years later, but it never came up. The whereabouts of the long lost son/brother was vaulted and perhaps that is how it should remain. I've heard that Bobby has had his ups and downs, but mostly ups. I am cautiously optimistic that he values his own future enough to nurture it.

That's the thing about being a doctor. You don't always get to hear the end of the story. People move. People die. People transfer their health care for a whole host of reasons. Medicine is a service profession. Doctors are here to serve, but doctors are people, too, and sometimes, they just want to know how the story ends.

Chapter Six

DON'T DIVE HEAD FIRST . . .

I hope I've been supportive
I've tried not to interfere
I never wanted to control you
With self-doubt or looming fear.

I ask though that you promise
This one request—don't negotiate
Because if you ignore my warning
Regret may come too late.

Never, Never dive head first
Into a pond, a pool, a lake.
A moment of lapsed judgment
Could mark a life's mistake.

To learn another way of living
It may be seemingly unfair
This will be your only choice
You'll live your life out in a chair.

The quadriplegics I have come to know
Have accessed inner strength
But to reverse their injury
They'd go to any length.

These folks have touched my life
To see their struggles of each day
To function in the world we know
In their unique and altered way.

Their strength and perseverance
An inspiration to us all
It seems our inconveniences
Through *their* eyes seem so small.

So please just heed my warning
In your mind you'll hear my voice
I don't care whose doing what nearby
Please make the only choice.

Don't dive head first . . .

***

I will never forget one of my first encounters with a quadriplegic patient. We knew in advance about his condition because the referring doctor had called me ahead of time and apprised me of some of his special medical needs. The patient himself had also mentioned his disability when making the appointment to ensure that he could access the office. The wheelchair ramp was assembled and the staff was anticipating his arrival. Nothing went as predicted after that, and I quickly accepted that I was not in charge of this visit.

First, he arrived alone. He rang on his cell phone and asked that someone open the door. Assumption number one was that he would have an able-bodied shadow of sorts with him to do mundane things like open the door or ring the doorbell. The receptionist hopped up quickly after receiving his cell phone call and, embarrassed, opened the door while apologizing for his need to wait outside while phoning us, sitting six feet away on the sidewalk. Graciously, he said it was no problem and that he was grateful for the human receptionist because phone trees posed a unique inconvenience for him.

Once inside he settled into the lobby, deftly maneuvering his chair. The receptionist reached for the clipboard containing the "new patient" information and stopped herself just before she handed him the clipboard and pen.

Registering new patients in the office had become a well-choreographed dance for her and this time, she was off the music. She stopped awkwardly and held the clipboard and pen close to her chest instead and said something on the order of, "We usually ask that new patients fill out this information sheet and sign the HIPAA (Health Insurance Portability and Accountability Act) privacy form on their initial visit. Would you like help with this?"

He accepted and she took a seat beside him in the lobby un-buffered by her receptionist's partition. He invited her into his personal space, asking that she find his wallet in his briefcase and locate his insurance card. Step by step, he reassured her that yes, it was okay for her to open his bag, and yes, he wanted her to flip open his wallet, bypassing his wedding picture, flipping past his visa, and locating his insurance information. And yes, putting it back when she finished copying it would be fine.

We were so concerned before his arrival that we would ensure his comfort and ironically, he spent much of the encounter ensuring that we were at ease. By the end of his registration process, the receptionist was no longer flustered. They even exchanged a chuckle or two and she announced to the nurse that he was ready to come back.

Once settled in the exam room with vital signs taken and introductions made, the nurse handed me the chart and said, "He's not on disability. He has commercial insurance."

Our office visit began with the usual platitudes and niceties. I remember entering the exam room and reflexively extending my hand for a shake. In an uncontrolled and zigzagging motion he reached his clubbed and contracted hand to me and I eventually clutched his unfeeling wrist in some awkward gesture of greeting. I made a mental note that he has no reasonable use of his fingers or hands. They remained perpetually clasped as if they once held a sheet of paper without the use of his opposing thumbs. It was the same hand gesture I will sometimes make with my newly painted fingernails, blowing on them to hasten the drying process. I took my place on my wheeled stool and positioned myself where we could be eye to eye. The nurse had earlier removed the patient's designated armchair to make room for his somewhat cumbersome electric wheelchair. The exam room was small as is befitting most doctors' offices nowadays, a product of cost-containment accomplished by lowering overhead expenses. I fired off my standard history taking questions and he answered them expertly.

I couldn't help but notice how neatly parted and combed his hair was—almost in a boyish cut reminiscent of a well-coiffed school photo. He had straight, white teeth and a warm smile. A green sweater vest and brown corduroys completed the conservative look with a thick black safety strap interrupting the creases on his pants securing his motionless legs to the chair. Big, black, shapeless orthopedic shoes (a size thirteen would have been my guess) were planted symmetrically on the foot rest, placed there no doubt by the same person who had fastened the safety belt across his legs.

I delayed acknowledgement of his disability in an attempt to normalize the visit. But looking back, that willful denial was probably to protect my own sensibilities more than to shield him from discussion of the obvious. He had already learned a new way of living. It was I who was being taught to navigate this new encounter.

After completing the routine questions, he asked me to locate a small photo album he had brought with him. He coaxed me through a search of his personal belongings the same manner he had just twenty minutes earlier with the receptionist. It became clear to me that he had grown accomplished at leading virtual strangers into and out of his personal space. After all, the simplest tasks require the assistance of others when you're numb from the nipples down, and thick, vinyl straps buckle you in place across the chest and shins respectively.

"Go ahead and open that book up. I want to introduce you to someone." The initial photo was a posed wedding shot. "That's me and Vera." The shot revealed a Barbie and Ken type of couple with pearly whites who no doubt were following expert instructions on pose and stance from an artistic wedding photographer. "We've recently celebrated fifteen years together," he remarked proudly. "Now that's a family picnic. We were married five years here. Ben's three years old there and Lilly's nine months." I did the pointing as he narrated the pictures.

Pretty, blonde Vera in Jackie "O" sunglasses stood with Lilly at her hip fussing with the bonnet strap under her chin. In another shot, the patient smiled as he was called to the camera while applying suntan lotion to Ben's freckled nose. Both wore matching swim trunks enjoying their July day in the sun. We flipped more pages and with each one I was introduced to more members of the extended family: two brothers similar to him in stature—tall, with sandy brown hair; and his mom, who was then still alive with an oversized straw hat and whiter than natural legs which she kept away from the sun ever since the doctor told her that sun exposure was to blame for those pesky age spots.

The last shot was of a young Jamaican woman with a soft smile and big black eyes posing at a kitchen table, her chin in her hands with her fingertips cupping her high cheekbones.

"This is Penelope. Penny for short. She's a member of my family now. Those summer photos were taken the day of my accident. At first, they were hard to look at. An hour after these shots were taken, my life changed forever. My family's life changed forever. It was a really nice summer day and we have lots of pictures to show for it. The photos just leave out me being airlifted out of my cousin's backyard, my four-week hospital stay and my four months at the spinal cord injury rehabilitation center. I bring this photo album when I want to introduce myself wholly to someone. I feel like you can't begin to know me now unless you've seen a little of me then. And since that day in July ten years ago, there's been an addition to my family—that's Penny." He chuckled and said, "Penny and I have had many an intimate moment. My wife never expected she'd have to share me with another woman. She probably never expected a lot of things."

There was a thick silence as he took a second to take a breath and shift in his chair, and I, with painstaking concentration, inspected a crack in my floor tile.

"There's a lot that goes into maintaining this appearance," he continued with a wide smile, inviting a chuckle from me and permission to continue the office visit with his disability acknowledged but not spotlighted.

I came to find out that he and his brothers own an insurance company and I politely nodded as he tried to educate me about the ins and outs of the business. As I've said before, I owe a lot of knowledge acquisition to my patient interactions, but some jobs I just don't understand no matter how many times folks share their work experiences with me. (Mergers and acquisitions is another, but I will keep trying to be receptive!)

His brothers have made adjustments in their work schedules so that he can come in later on Tuesdays and Fridays.

"I have a date with Penny every Tuesday and Friday morning for my bowel protocol. I don't get to work 'til eleven a.m. on those days, but I'll argue that I'm less full of shit than my brothers!" He really was so witty that you couldn't help but laugh in spite of yourself at what probably were not "PC" jokes. But I suppose that when a quadriplegic makes a joke about his own bowel regimen, it's ok to laugh if it was funny.

All jokes aside, the simplest tasks require preparation, planning, and the assistance of others for someone with this kind of disability. It is unfathomable to me to have to wait for my teeth to be brushed or my hair to be combed or a tear to be wiped away. He tells me that he's learned a new way of living. He meaningfully and irreplaceably contributes to his family as a husband, father, and provider.

Despite his apparent poise and strength, there has to be regret. There has to be a mourning of the accident anniversary each summer or a sting of envy as he watches his brother throw a ball with his son while he cheers them on from his perch in the shade. (Quadriplegics have trouble with thermoregulation so overheating in the sun can be quite dangerous.)

If he had those raw feelings, he spared me them. As I watched his high-backed wheelchair narrowly clear the door hinges as he approached the exit, I couldn't help but think, "Don't dive head first."

On the way out of the office that day, we noticed that he didn't park in the driveway, but on the street. We let him know that he could park in the driveway parking lot closer to the entrance in the future. He answered, "That's ok. What if an older person needs to park there? After all, I'm on wheels."

***

It is difficult to render me speechless, but I recall standing silently, a guest in my own lobby, as I watched him scoot down the ramp and on to the sidewalk toward his souped-up car. He left a humbled, thoughtful staff in his wake.

I channel my experience with him when perspective is called for; like when a dad at a fifth grade back to school night asks how the teachers plan to prepare children for the academic rigors of high school. Or when a swim coach explains that swim team is a six day a week commitment and that the Saturday meets would need to supersede all family and friend gatherings whether it be a milestone grandparent birthday or a close friend's dance recital.

I especially reflect on my encounter when I see a perfectly able-bodied woman in a fur fedora and matching fur-trimmed snow boots hop out of her SUV after peeling into the handicapped parking space just to run a quick errand. In truth, it makes me want to key the car or at the very least, call the ASPCA.

I could run sentence into sentence mistaking length for persuasiveness, but I'll try not to. Of course, first and foremost, I'd like to admonish everyone by saying, "Don't dive head first," but perhaps the softer undercurrent of my advice is, "Don't take ability for granted." May you never be the woman in the fur-trimmed fedora or the man who hangs the handicapped parking sticker from his car visor long after the death of his mother, the original holder of the placard. May you never aspire to mediocrity when excellence is in reach and may you never cocoon yourself too snuggly in the soft throw of self-pity while a prize slips narrowly from your grasp. When I see the wet eyes of failed attempts or hear the huffs of frustrated tries, I say that I once knew a man who couldn't move his arms or legs, who never considered himself disabled, and who, in the face of adversity, was still able to put the needs of others before his own. Nothing dries an eye or hushes a huff faster.

Chapter Seven

A DOE-EYED LADY

Much like a volcano
Erupting unpredictably
Sloppy and erratic
Such pain is difficult to see

It's not for me to watch and judge
To note how some folks can achieve
A dignified and noble peace
A graceful way to grieve.

There once was a doe-eyed lady
Elegant, well-read
She'd lost a lot of weight by then
Eyes, too big for her head

She'd raised three boys to mighty heights
They stood in silent strength
To see their mom in less distress
They'd go to any length.

But no words need be spoken
Quiet, thoughtful – they were worn
It wasn't now for them to speak
A touching way to mourn.

It wasn't time for them to claim
The center spot on stage
It was about their mother now
Giving in to her old age.

She said, "My life has been dismantled,
But I find myself still here.
I am not one to overstay
The time to go is near."

Gnarled fingers like tree branches
Arthritic in their bend
Wrapped around her one son's wrist
She knew that it was near the end.

A warm and tired smile
A look that said, "I know."
She nodded to her boys above
A peaceful letting go.

***

I had just opened my office and there weren't too many
patients on the roster yet. My receptionist at the time, Katie,
would pick up the silent phone receiver and stage whisper,
"Hello? Hello?" and then hang it up while saying loudly enough
for me to hear, "Just checking that we have a dial tone!" Her
contagious giggle rippled down the empty corridor to my office

as I thumbed through the local doctor registry looking for the next "meet and greet" victim. I could only stomach three "meet and greets" in a day so I tried to be strategic about the type and location of doctors in the community to meet. We had no highway billboards or radio minutes advertising the office, so hoofing it with a stack of business cards in my pocket was the best way to let colleagues know that we were open. I cringe a little when I think of the "meet and greet." It's an absolutely brutal experience if you're not a natural salesperson and even if you are, selling oneself leaves a slimy trail in one's wake no matter how graciously the pitch is executed. I'd idle outside an office and convince myself to go in with the taciturn agreement that I'd be able to share the exchange with Katie afterwards in the car. She had one of those infectious, bubbly laughs that made you, as the storyteller, want to be funny just so you could hear it. That dynamic largely defined our relationship—me, the animated storyteller and Katie, the ever-receptive, enthusiastic listener. This exchange propelled us through the first three years of my practice's start-up. Her laughter invigorated me and I can only hope that it was always as heartfelt as it was robust.

Most of the time, my colleagues were compassionate about the painful introduction and politely took my not too thick, not too thin stack of business cards. I'd pre-secured them with a rubber band for ease of hand off and to avoid the potential cascade of twenty cards to the ground should the delicately choreographed end of meeting handshake go awry. I'd conclude the encounter, get back in the car, and call the office from my mobile phone. The phone rang once and I'd hear on the other end.

"How did it go?" Katie asked.

"Now was that the script?" I answered.

"Oh sorry, I saw your name on the caller ID. Do you want me to start again?"

"Yes. Please," I said, smiling to myself.

"Good morning. Dr. Holt's office. This is Katie speaking. How may I help you?" she said.

"Fabulous! You sound very welcoming," I reassured.

"Why thank you. So, how did it go?"

I was thrilled that Katie had such a "happy voice" and was sure that this had to win over some patients more than the dreaded computer-generated one that marched the caller through a series of phone prompts. This live person on the other end had to matter for something, I'd say to myself, given that medicine is a service profession after all.

"How did what go?" I asked.

"Oh my gosh! The meet and greet?!"

"Let me start by saying, it was weird," I reported succinctly. And there was that giggle again—an invitation to continue with the story. "Now, Katie, you don't mind if I first go through my recitation?"

"Of course not. Go ahead," she encouraged solemnly.

Staring blankly out of the car window as I idled in the parking lot, I said aloud,

"It was very nice of him to meet with me. I'm so glad that I had the opportunity to introduce myself. No one's going to know we're open if I'm just sitting in a suburban office picking at my cuticles." I concluded my recitation monotonously and would say this over and over to myself in one form or another as I tried to keep up my "meet and greet" momentum.

"That's right. Absolutely no cuticle picking," Katie affirmed.

I sighed a theatrical exhale and said, "Where do I begin? Perhaps I'll start with the waft of hazelnut coffee brew that assaulted my nose upon office entry with the trickle of the waterfall to my right and the aquarium straight ahead with a discrete sign discouraging anyone from feeding the fish."

"No!"

"Yes. I was in a plastic surgeon's office after all. And did I mention the sign?"

"No. What sign?"

"The one that said, 'you are what you eat and you can put it on your face.'"

"What?" she sputtered and began her noiseless laughing. If you didn't know better, you'd be tempted to ask, "Katie? Kate? Are you there?" But just when you began to worry, you'd hear her catch her breathe and burst into giggles.

As I was sure she was reaching for tissues to dab the corners of her eyes (Katie was a wet-eyed laughter), I said again, for effect and repeated for additional clarity,

"Yes. The sign read, 'you are what you eat and you can put it on your face.' So, Katie, the next time you reach for that pop tart, consider smearing the gooey insides on your nose to clean your pores. Or better yet, take some cheese wiz on a saltine, smash it on your eyes, and *voila*! No more dark circles!"

Choking back tears, Katie said, "I will consider this. So, I guess there wasn't a love connection?"

"I don't think we'll be referring patients back and forth to one another if that's what you mean, but he was reasonably nice. I left him cards and I have his here too—no jelly or mustard stains so he must keep them separate from the facials. Anyway, that's how things went with me. How about you? Anything exciting?"

"Well, yes, we got a bite. A nice older lady who said that her son sent her. She relocated to the area recently and she saw your brochure in her building."

"Uggh," I groaned. "That brochure is so dreadful."

"No, it is not. And it worked because she's coming in later in the week. Oops, the other line's ringing, gotta go." She hung up. I was left to buff up my ego alone in the car as I plugged the next meet and greet address into the GPS.

Katie and I made it to the end of the week without too many trials and tribulations. She'd managed to schedule four patients for Friday, which was grounds for a firework celebration in those days.

Friday came and in walked a darling older woman. Her hair was touched up an unnatural shade of dark brown that had a purple hue in our fluorescent lighting, and her eyes were wide-set and dark reminding me of the Betty Boop cartoon character. She came armed with a stack of medical files, a hard-covered book, and a wicker purse like the one Dorothy carried Toto in. After making the introductions with Katie, she took a seat in the lobby chair closest to the doors. Everyone took a seat in that chair, which would later explain why we had to rotate it with the other eleven waiting room chairs over six months and why the legs' spokes were so firmly indented in the carpet that not even professional cleaning could smooth them. Katie processed her paperwork and motioned to Marion that she was ready.

"My, you don't even let the seat get warm in this place. How's a girl to get any reading done?" Marion asked.

"No rest for you. Come on back. Do you need help carrying anything?" Katie asked, leaning forward with an extended hand ready to grab something.

"No, I don't need help. Do I seem this infirm to you? You're just like my son, God love him. 'Mom, don't lift that. Mom, I got that.' I've got everything. Just show me the way." She smiled widely and remarkably her eyes didn't squint at all. They remained as round and open as a doll's no matter what the rest of her face was doing.

"Very good. Follow me," Katie instructed and she led her into the exam room. "Can I take those files from you and make copies so I can show them to the doctor?"

"No need for copies, dear. I don't have much use for the gibberish in there. Maybe she does. Consider those yours."

"Thanks, I'll take them."

"I take it that my seat won't get very warm in here either?"

she said, fingering her bookmark deciding whether it would be worthwhile to open to the saved page.

"Nope. No warm seats in here either. She'll be right in," Katie said, excusing herself and exiting the exam room.

In those days, our punctuality was more easily achieved. I've always been a stickler for timeliness and I try to this day to stick closely to the day's schedule. Fortunately, Katie was the same way and running too behind made her uncomfortably anxious, so there weren't many warm seats.

"Good morning," I said, motioning to Marion to stay seated. "No need to get up on my account. I hope you're well."

"As well as can be expected at my age, I suppose."

"What age?" I said in mock surprise.

"Oh honey, please. Didn't they teach you to read the chart before you see a patient? Look at that birth date. Horrifying really."

"Well, you look great," I reassured.

"Thanks," she said, cocking her chin up at me slightly, letting me know that I was on notice and that future flattery would get me nowhere. I rolled my wheeled stool in her direction and began squeezing the excess air out of the blood pressure cuff.

"I just want to check your blood pressure. Do you have a favorite arm?"

"Anyone you'd like," she offered both up in front of her and started to push up the baggy sleeve.

"Don't bunch it all up. I'll probably be able to listen through the fabric," I said as I wrapped the cuff around her narrow arm. "My, you're a skinny one," I remarked, trying to fasten the far edge of the Velcro together so that the cuff didn't just slide off.

"Isn't it always that way? You diet all your young life to maintain a girlish figure and now all I want to do is put weight on—but not here," she said as she patted a rather protuberant belly.

"It is a funny thing, isn't it?" I acknowledged and began inflating the cuff.

"Has your belly always been this distended?" I asked, putting the stethoscope to my ears. "Hold on a minute. Don't answer yet," and I let the dial tick down in numbers until I heard her systolic at eighty-eight followed by her diastolic number at fifty-eight. "88/58," I said out loud, unplugging my ears and turning my attention back to Marion. "As we were saying. Has your belly always been this pooched out?"

She furrowed her brow.

"It's a medical term—distended?"

She smiled in return and said, "I actually had quite a nice shape in my day, but over the last three years, I've lost weight in my arms and legs. Look how spindly they are," demonstrating by flicking the excess fabric around her biceps. "And my stomach has gotten huge. It's impossible to dress a figure like this, I assure you."

"Well, again you look great." Her furrowed brow and raised chin silently urged me to rein it in. "Good?" I asked seeking her approval.

"I'll take good out of politeness' sake," she said.

"Your blood pressure's a bit low, but I guess it's high enough for you. Do you feel ok?"

"Yes. Oh gosh, I'm fine. I don't know what all the fuss is about. I'm widowed seven years by now and my sons were absolutely insistent that I move up here closer to them. What do they think I did before they were born? How do they suppose I managed?"

"It comes from a good place, I'm sure. They just want you in arm's reach should you need anything," I reassured.

"Oh, I know. I have good boys. You know my oldest, I think he and his wife come here too."

"I believe that they do," I nodded, wheeling back to the exam table where I was taking notes in her chart. "So has this belly distension been investigated before you moved here, by your other doctors, I mean?"

"Oh yes, with countless tests. It even got rock-hard once, and I had a lot of pain. I ended up at the local hospital. That's when my granddaughter decided I had ovarian cancer," she said matter of factly.

"Oh? Is she in medicine?" I asked.

"No, she's in hair. She's a beautician, but she's addicted to that darn computer like so many other kids her age. She sent my son into a tailspin telling him that I had all the symptoms of ovarian cancer and that the end was probably near."

"And that wasn't true?" I asked. My initial appraisal of her symptoms—weight loss, abdominal distension—was leading me to a similar conclusion.

"No it wasn't true. It turns out that that pain I was having was a twisted bowel or something, like an obstruction," she explained.

"And what caused that?" I asked, pen in hand since this spunky lady seemed more well versed in her health affairs than one might have initially thought.

"Well, two things. They say I have malabsorption and short bowel syndrome."

"Hmmm." I scribbled this down.

"Do you get taught to make that sound in medical school?"

"What sound? Hmmm?" I said again, this time cupping my chin in my hand stroking a mock beard.

"Yes, hmmm," she echoed, mirroring back the beard stroking motion which appeared even more exaggerated with her skinny, long fingers.

"Maybe. It's a trade secret. If I tell you, I'd have to kill you and that would be bad for my image, you know?" I said.

"Of course. The doctors said 'Hmmm' a lot when I was first hospitalized for my digestive issues. They delicately said that certain gastrointestinal disorders are often detected in a younger patient—at least 'on initial presentation' to borrow a doctor term. So I puzzled them. I think that my granddaughter was both relieved and silently disappointed that she couldn't crack the case on the Internet," she explained.

"I'm glad she wasn't right."

"Me too, dear."

The office visit concluded with Marion saying that it was "hot as blazes" out and it was nice that her fifty-five-and-older condominium complex had a communal pool.

"Not that I relish putting on a swimsuit with this physique, but I have no one to impress at my age," she asserted. "They call it fifty-five-and-older, but it's really seventy-five and older by the looks of things, so I fit in pretty well there at eighty-five years young."

"I'm glad that you're adjusting, Marion. Moving is hard. Keep us posted on how you're getting along."

"Oh I will, and if I don't, Douglas will, I'm sure." Marion mentioning her son's name made me reflect on his recent "to establish" office visit in my mind's eye. It's always intriguing to see two and three generations of the same family in the office, but it's particularly puzzling to me how such solid, strapping men—some even imposing in stature—can come from such delicate, little moms. I wonder if mothers of sons muse about the same thing as they drop their boys off at college and then retrieve them four years later as young men?

The next time we saw Marion, it was a little after Halloween and she came into the office to receive her flu shot. Katie roomed her, took her vital signs, and was making small talk as I drew the flu shot up in the lab area. I heard Katie laughing through the closed door saying,

"Marion, these are great! Oh will you look at this one? And who's this?" Marion, more muffled by the closed door could not be heard well, but she was animatedly talking Katie through a series of photographs. "Ok, she'll be right in," Katie said. "Keep those out 'cause I know she'll want to see them."

Juggling the flu shot, alcohol pad, band-aid, and chart in one hand, I managed to knock and open the door to find Marion smiling to herself flipping through a plastic photo album.

"Hi there," I announced. "I heard you and Katie laughing. What have you got?" I asked, freeing my hands setting the whole pile of things on the exam table. I took my blue stool and glided over to her. She nudged her chair closer to me, but without wheels, it didn't move much. Assuring her that I could see, I craned my neck to share in her happiness.

"There was a Halloween party at my apartment complex. At first I wasn't going to go but then I said to myself, 'Marion, you can sit in your one bedroom apartment and sulk the rest of your life away or you can get to it!'"

"That seems like the right approach. Congratulations," I commented.

"Thank you," she said with satisfaction. "That's me," she clarified, pointing with her bony finger. Her orange wig was a cross between that of Anne of Green Gables and Pippi Longstocking and I remember thinking that the orange was a little unnatural, but suited her perfectly. She had inked some strategic freckles over her cheeks and had tied checkered bows at the bottom of her braids. "I'm Raggedy Anne. And see that?" she said gesturing again with her knobby finger.

"Yes."

"She's Minnie Pearl. Do you see the price tag hanging off her hat?"

"I do." Fortunately, I was old enough to remember Minnie Pearl, but if I were ten years younger, she would have lost me.

"And this fellow was a strip of bacon and see that there on his chest?" she asked.

I squinted to try to make it out. "Something's taped on the

costume, right?" I asked.

"Yes, it's his bottle of cholesterol medication. Get it? His cholesterol medication is taped over his heart as he's wearing a bacon costume—really very clever, I thought."

I chuckled and nodded. "Yes, it really was. It seems like there's a nice group of people in your place. I'm so glad you're doing well."

"Yes, there really are lovely folks there and the ones who aren't, you just can't notice them. I thought you'd get a kick out of these." She stuffed the photo album into her purse. I remember being happy that it was so compact that she could carry it with her. This way, she'd always have a reason to smile to herself.

"I'll take that signed consent form," I said, reaching for it and attaching it to her chart. "Let's give you this flu shot."

She was already wriggling her arm out of her floppy sweater exposing her bony shoulder.

"Is it possible that you're thinner?" I asked, cleaning her upper arm with alcohol preparing the area for her shot.

"In all the wrong places, maybe. I eat. I really do. I just go slow. You know, small portions and frequent meals."

"That's good. Small pinch," I said almost simultaneously with the injection.

"You're good at that."

"First time," I responded walking the needle over to the red sharps container. "Why don't we weigh you," I suggested and she was already stepping out of her laceless loafers and walking in her stocking feet over to the scale. "One hundred and five, give or take," I pronounced and jotted it in the chart while at the same time, noting that she was one hundred nine pounds three months ago. "You'll have to be careful. You're down four pounds. It could be nothing, but you should be aware."

"I know, dear. I'm certainly not trying to lose any more. I don't want my face to appear gaunt." I didn't have the heart to tell her that her face was already gaunt, so I was grateful that her perception of herself was more forgiving.

"Have you been having abdominal pain?" I probed. Marion was an "under-reporter." Everything was always "just fine really," or it was, "absolutely nothing," or at other times she just "didn't know what all the fuss was about." A doctor is obligated to do the asking with an "under-reporter."

"Not much," she answered slipping her feet back in her shoes balancing with one hand on the armrest of the patient chair.

"What's not much?"

"It's not really pain?"

"If it's not pain, then what is it?"

"I'd call it discomfort."

"Ok. So have you been having any discomfort?" I asked with mock exaggeration.

"Some."

"Where?"

"Here," she said, gesturing to her protuberant belly button. I poked it with my finger watching the outie become an innie under the pressure of my touch and right itself as an outie again with my release.

"Like the Pillsbury Dough boy commercial," I remarked.

"Wonderful," she said.

"Seriously. If your pain—I mean discomfort—increases in frequency, I need you to call. Don't just let it progress, ok Marion?"

"Ok."

"So call if anything worsens."

"Ok."

"Fine." I washed my hands and pulled my industrial-strength brown towelettes out of the container. "Do you need anything else?" I asked, discarding my crumpled paper towel.

"No, dear. I'm fine and I will call if I need anything."

"Ok, Marion. Behave yourself," I admonished as I exited the exam room.

"That's no fun," she answered, gathering her belongings to leave.

Not too many weeks went by before I got a Saturday morning call from Douglas. All of my patients have my cell phone number, but you'd be surprised how few of them use it.

"Doctor Elaine?" he asked, not expecting me to answer, but rather a service operator.

"Yes."

"Oh great. I'm glad it's you. This is Douglas. I'm calling about my mom."

"What's wrong with Marion?"

"Well, it started about four days ago. At first she was having twinges in her stomach."

"Where?" I asked.

"Where mom?" he asked away from the receiver. He evidently was calling me from her apartment and I could only assume that it wasn't a good sign that she wasn't coming to the phone herself.

"She said around the belly button." I heard her muffled words in the background and Douglas clarified, "But they were just twinges then. Now she seems kind of worse off. Her belly is even more distended and she says it's rock hard. And . . . what's that mom?" he asked directing his attention away from the phone. "Ok, I'll tell her. She says she's terribly nauseous too now."

"Shoot," I said. "Douglas, it sounds like we could be getting into trouble again with her bowel. I'm afraid that I have no choice but to direct you to the emergency room. I will call over there and tell them to expect you. Will you be able to drive your mother or will you be calling EMS?"

"I don't know. Mom, do you think you can get into my car? No, I don't have the truck. I have the sedan. Ok, ok I will."

I held on through this exchange, mentally scheduling my afternoon, seeing as I would likely end up in the emergency room at some point later in the day.

"Doctor?"

"Yep."

"I'll drive mom over to the emergency room now."

"Ok. I'll call over there and tell them to expect you. Please use my name when you arrive, and they'll call me once they've got some tests back."

"Alright. That's what we'll do. Thanks. And mom's saying thank you, too."

"No problem. Tell her I'll see her later."

"Will do. See you later." Douglas hung up.

It would be a few hours before the ER staff had any test results back so I itinerated my Saturday errands and gathered up the dry cleaning. I always kept a stethoscope in my glove compartment and my hospital ID badge in my wallet so that if the ER called and I was close to the hospital, I could just swing by in between stops. As suspected, Marion's bowel condition had worsened and the emergency room doctor was concerned that she would need surgery. I rattled off the name of the surgeon I wanted consulted and said that I'd be over that way soon.

When I arrived, the ER buzzed with its characteristic dynamic chaos. Gurneys lined hallways and those patients lying on hospital stretchers in the corridors enviously watched the patients who had earned themselves actual exam rooms. I had called ahead of time and learned that Marion was in room five, subverting my need to ask the ER staff for any directions. I beelined to room five, stethoscope, car keys, ID badge, and pen in hand to see Douglas' long legs crossed, peeking out from the edge of the drawn curtain. His over-sized docksider was tapping the air nervously and I stopped briefly outside of the curtain to listen for their conversation.

Taking the silence as my cue to enter, I snuck around the curtain and said,

"Fancy seeing you both here."

Douglas half-stood to reach my extended hand as he closed a heavy looking hard-covered book. "And you, Miss. I thought I told you to behave yourself?" I said, turning toward Marion, who appeared as a caricature of her former self. A nasogastric tube was secured into one nostril with white paper tape as the other end of the tubing extended to a wall suction unit. A putrid, viscous liquid was being pumped into a clear canister. Liquidy, brown bubbles traveled from her nose to the wall unit through the plastic tubing like a mouse might travel through the digestive tract of a python—with slow, steady, peristaltic motion. It was hard not to wince at her obvious discomfort and as I turned my attention to Marion extending my hand to her, she feebly lifted her hand to meet mine. Our handshake melted into a hold as she allowed her arm to drift back down on the stretcher.

I kept my hand in her grasp as she choked out, "If this is misbehaving, it's not worth it." Her words were garbled as she tried to project them around the tube in her throat. Swallowing was an effort, making her words moist with excess saliva.

"Don't try to talk. Those NG tubes are horrible and we hope that you won't have it in for long. Are you terribly uncomfortable now?" I asked.

"Not bad," she answered.

Douglas interjected, "She got morphine not too long ago, which seemed to help."

"Good." I took my stethoscope and tried to listen to her belly. It was indeed more protuberant than ever and her skin felt taut even through the hospital Johnny coat. I went to lift the gown a bit to expose her abdomen thinking that I might be able to listen better without the thin layer of clothes muffling her already distant, if not absent, bowel sounds. As I went to do so, Douglas shifted his chair so that his back faced us affording his mother privacy. I remember being touched by the discretion and subtlety of that gesture—such a simple and quiet display of modesty and respect even in the face of their changing child-parent roles. Ultimately, exposure of her bare belly to my stethoscope didn't help and indeed I could hear no bowel sounds.

"I'm afraid that this time your gut may not fix itself, Marion." Douglas was righting his chair by now so that the three of us could face each other during the explanation. "It would seem that you're obstructed. There's a blockage and it will either correct itself with bowel rest and observation or it will need to be surgically repaired," I explained.

"The emergency room physician said the same thing, so Mom and I have had time to talk about things. If surgery is ultimately what's needed, then that's what we'll do," said Douglas. Marion nodded in affirmation as continued talking with the NG tube in place had grown discouraging.

"Very well. That seems reasonable. We usually give it a day or two and then we start decision-making. You'll be meeting the surgeon soon and you should direct your surgical questions to him. Whenever we operate on someone eighty-something years young, there's always risk, but we may be given little choice in this scenario. Questions for me?" Marion shook her head slowly, careful not to dislodge the tube. Douglas said that they understood everything so far and that they would wait to see the surgeon and take things one day at a time. I told them to have the nurses reach out to me if anything came up and assured both Douglas and his mother that I'd be back in the morning to check on the progress of things. Marion mouthed a, "Thank you," and Douglas assured me that he'd call if there were any new developments. I exited the curtained room number five and they resumed the comfort of their silent communication. Douglas settled, book in hand, in his bedside chair and Marion gingerly repositioined her head on the crinkly, disposable pillow careful not to disturb the paper tape on her nose.

***

Marion made it through the surgery, but not without looking paler and seeming frailer. Just walking from the bed to the bathroom was a struggle. It was her fourth day in the hospital and her bowel had begun to gurgle and reawaken after the stun of anesthesia and surgery. I knocked before entering the room, but she seemed sound asleep sitting in the bedside chair. A breakfast tray served as a lap belt of sorts, holding her in her seat. I remember thinking that at least there would be a lot of noise when she keeled over into it, taking her Jell-o and clear liquid diet with her.

"Marion?" I said, tapping her claw hand as it rested on her lap. She stirred a bit, but kept her chin tucked into her chest. *This can't be comfortable*, I thought to myself and gently lifted her chin up, righting her head. That was enough to rouse her.

"Oh, you are an early bird, aren't you? I haven't even been able to wash my hair," she said, smoothing down the stray ends.

"You look maa'velous darling. How are you feeling?"

"Alright, I suppose, all things considered."

"How's the liquid diet?" I asked, motioning to the untouched breakfast tray.

"Well, I wouldn't recommend the green Jell-o. That is supposed to be lime, but it has an almost metallic taste to it. If you ever get the chance to choose, I advise the red or the orange."

"Good to know. It looks like we'll be able to spring you tomorrow if all continues to go well. Will you be going home or do you think you'll need a brief rehabilitation stay?" I asked.

"Oh no, dear. Home, please."

"That's fine. I was just giving you options."

"I know. My husband was in and out of rehabilitation centers towards the end. I'm familiar with the process, but I'd like to try to maintain my independence."

"I understand."

"Of course, I don't want to burden the children. Their lives are so busy, you know."

"I do. So let's try home tomorrow with visiting nurse and some additional help if you need? I'll give Douglas a ring and tell him the plan?"

"Yes, dear. Please give him a call so he can make arrangements. I hate to disrupt his day," she said as she began fiddling with the cellophane wrap on the jiggly Jell-o cubes.

"Do you need any help, Marion?" I asked as I prepared to leave.

"No. You run along and take care of sick people now. I'm really just fine." And she went about deconstructing the breakfast tray.

Marion transitioned home and followed up in the office after the hospital stay using a wheeled walker to assist her gait. It additionally had a mesh pouch for her belongings so she didn't burden her aide with requests to lug around her personal items. I was happy to see the corner of her small, plastic photo album peeking out of her handbag amidst a zip-lock bag full of pill bottles.

At the same time that Marion was recovering from her latest hospitalization, another patient of mine was convalescing from his in a rehabilitation center. I spent two afternoons a week in a physical rehabilitation center where I saw patients for an abbreviated period of time as they bridged a transition from hospital to home. These patients were too well for hospital care and too ill for home discharge. I was the "foster doctor" in a sense and provided temporary care before the patient was well enough to be packaged up and sent back to the original community doctor. The unsettling transition from hospital to rehab center combined with the fear of uncertain prognosis often caused the least attractive qualities in patients and their families to surface. At times, irritability and impatience brimmed close to a boil as visitors cared for their loved ones. Staff and doctors were always poised to deflect anger and to temper worry while addressing patient and family concerns. Like walking on a tight rope, it is both crazy and exhilarating.

A man was being wheeled on a stretcher trailed by his son, who carried personal belongings in white plastic bags. The son's overgrown beard and glad-bag satchels fashioned him an unlikely Santa Claus as he lumbered close to the stretcher awaiting directions from the transporting EMS workers. The form on the stretcher resembled neither man nor woman. He had no hair and no discernable eyelashes. His frame was delicate and contracted at the elbows, wrists, and knees in bird-like contortion and his head nestled neatly into the crook of his left clavicle as if he were flinching. The stretcher slowed at the nurse's station as the transporters waited for the room assignment. The unit clerk, with an ear to the phone, motioned to room 114, bed one, and the EMS worker nodded in acknowledgement.

The Santa son must not have recognized the wordless communication and approached the desk, bags in hand, and asked, "Where's my dad's room?"

"114. I just told the EMS guys. Just follow them," said the clerk. still on hold with the phone receiver to her ear.

"You hear that, daddy? We are going to room 114," said the son, leaning over the stretcher side rails. Truth be told, it was unclear if his father heard him, could understand him, or even cared.

"He's yours," the unit clerk whispered to me as she hung up the phone in frustration.

"Thanks," I whispered back knowingly.

I gave the EMS workers time to settle both father and son into the room and continued writing in the charts. When I saw them wheel the empty stretcher out and wish everyone at the desk a good day, I knew that I didn't have too much time before the son would reappear at the desk, advocating for his father's care needs. Preempting that scene, I gathered my stethoscope, phone, pen, and paper and headed into room 114. The son was bent over the bedside drawers unloading his dad's personal belongings and I knocked, careful not to startle him.

"Sir? I'm one of the doctors here at the facility, and I want to introduce myself to you and your father."

"Oh, ok. Come in," he answered as he scuttled to his feet. "I was just putting some of my dad's things away. His electric razor, his dentures, and some books."

I looked over at his father as he said this. His books? I thought to myself. Does this son think his father's going to read these? The man doesn't turn his head or move his limbs? No one's joining the book club anytime soon.

Just as I finished this internal narrative, the son said:

"I read to him every night. It helps him fall asleep." My thought bubble read: *Shame on you, Elaine!* With a wagging finger if those can be included in a thought bubble.

"Of course. Don't let me interrupt you. I already know a little about your father from the hospital chart. How long has he been bed bound?" I asked.

"Oh, he's not bedbound. He loves car rides, especially with the windows down."

"Really? Was he more mobile before the hospital stay?" The son looked at me kind of confused and didn't answer, so I thought I'd rephrase the question. "Was he walking and getting around better before he went into the hospital?"

"Well, no. He had his stroke six years ago and he's been pretty much like this. He went into the hospital because of a urinary infection," the son explained.

"I thought I'd heard that. So how do you get him into the car for your rides?"

"I carry him," he said matter of factly, and I pictured a prehistoric scene with a person's body petrified in a fixed shape slung over the shoulder of an ambling caveman. I nodded contemplatively and the son thankfully interjected before I could muster up a reply. "Are there special visiting hours here?"

"I think that the staff is flexible about it. Why do you ask?"

"Because I have to read to him at night. I had to leave the hospital by eight p.m., but that was a little early."

"I think that you can stay later than that if you'd like."

"Oh, good. You know, I've been taking care of him for the last six years. The house is lonely without him. We have to get him home soon," he said, stroking his father's bare forehead.

I was able to move fairly quickly through the physical exam. I found myself altering my questions to his doting son treading gently on what seemed like fragile sensibilities.

"Now, has Dad always been this thin?"

"You think he's too thin?" the son asked almost panicked.

The contour of his dad's face had begun to resemble a biology class skull with all the subcutaneous fat gone except for the loose jowl below his chin. His xyphoid process and rib edges were so prominent that his stomach appeared concave even when you propped him up into a sitting position. Yet, in spite of this, the burly Santa son seemed surprised at the observation that his father was underweight?

"I'm sure that he's had trouble eating since the stroke, right? He probably only eats soft foods?" I asked, eye-averting the son and focused instead on tucking his father under the covers concluding my physical exam.

"Yeah, he does. Sometimes I even blend the food up and give it to him with a straw. He sips real good from a straw. This way it's less messy too. You may want to tell the folks here that that's how he likes it. Do you want me to?" And he motioned to get up from his chair with the intent of heading to the front desk with his straw revelation.

"You can stay here with your dad. I'm heading back up front and I'll be sure to let the speech pathologist and the nutritionist know about your concerns." He stared back at me, not entirely satisfied that I'd follow through with my task, coercing me to reassure him. "Truly. I promise. I will tell them about the blended food and the straws. I will also order that he have assistance with all his meals so that you don't have to worry when you're not here."

I gathered my things and planned to head out when he stopped me and said, "You're going to take care of him right? We've got to get him home as soon as he's better. It's just him and me at home, right, Dad?" he said, reaching for his father's contracted arm.

"We'll get him better and back home," I reassured and told him that I would be back within the next few days to check on his father's progress. That seemed to please him and I concluded the encounter no more certain about how these two were managing at home than when I'd started.

Upon my arrival at the front desk, I dutifully gave the "straw" feedback to both the nutritionist and speech pathologist who made a note of it.

I additionally handed the unit clerk the orders for admission blood work and assisted feedings and in return, she asked: "What's up there?"

"Up where?"

"Room 114. Something seems off."

"Oh right. Well, a doting son who seems to care, but he may not get it, you know?"

"Yeah something's funny."

"Well, I trust your instincts, Miss Fran, so I'll keep my eyes open."

"You do that, and I'll do the same."

"Deal. Call me if you need anything. I'll see you Thursday."

"Will do," she said, faxing the medication orders to the pharmacy.

Back at the office, Katie had just received a call. It was Douglas. He said that his mother's stomach was distended and hurting again and he was heading to her place to take her to the emergency room. She'd only been home for a brief while this time and it seemed that the interval between episodes was shortening. If I had that "here we go again" feeling, Marion must have been even more exasperated. By the time I reached the ER, she already had her NG tube inserted and putrid, gastric contents were being forced into the wall suction unit tube. This time, Douglas paced outside the exam room fiddling with his phone in search of reception.

I startled him when I came up behind him and said, "We meet again."

"Oh, hi Doc. Yeah, we love you but we'd like to stop meeting like this. I was jus trying to reach my wife. It looks like we're admitting mom again. Another small bowel obstruction," he said, resigned to the fact that he wasn't going to get cell phone service and clipped the useless phone to his belt loop.

"My friend, I'm sorry we're here again," I said, entering the exam room.

"Me too," she mouthed back unable to speak with any kind of audible volume.

"Are you in a lot of pain?"

Douglas answered, "They just gave her some morphine."

"Good stuff," Marion whispered and winked.

"Ok, as long as you're comfortable for now. You know the routine. I'll call the surgeon. We'll get serial films and we'll hope your gut rights itself."

She forced a smile and closed her eyes allowing her tired head to bob forward. Her gray roots were coming in, accentuating her middle part. It made me sad to see the fade of her dark, purple-brown hair.

"Douglas, I'm going to push paper and get her up to her bed on the floor. We'll take it one day at a time," I said. We both took a moment to watch Marion sleep propped up in her hospital gurney.

I gathered my keys and stethoscope to leave when Douglas said without averting his eyes from his sleeping mother, "Thanks Doc. I'll be here."

She narrowly escaped the need for surgery, but five days without eating or getting out of bed had significantly weakened the already feeble Marion.

"You'll get out of bed and sit in the chair today, ok Marion?"

"Wow. Now that's excitement," she answered.

"Don't underestimate the energy that that's going to expend. It will be good to get moving. It will help your bowels reawaken."

"Then, sit in a chair, I will," she affirmed.

"I'm glad we could avoid surgery this time."

"You and me both. But frankly, I don't think I would have done it."

"You don't think you would have done what?"

"The surgery. I don't think that I would have gone through with it."

"I know that you're weak, but I think you could have survived another surgery. I think you would have made it, I mean."

"Maybe. Maybe not. I just don't think that's what I would have done. It's my decision, you know," she said, standing her ground.

"Of course," I affirmed. "You are guiding this ship. I just want to make sure that you understand that if a bowel obstruction turns out to be stubborn enough that surgery is the only way to repair it, to decline surgery would mean an inevitable worsening of your condition."

"Oh, will you stop dancing around. If I ran into real trouble and decided not to have the surgery, I would die," she translated.

"Possibly, yes," I acknowledged.

"You have to put the 'possibly' in there. Always hedging your bets, you doctors are," she said in mock exasperation.

"Ok, Miss, so let's sit in the chair today and have physical therapy work with you a bit. I know that you've wanted to avoid rehabilitation center stays in the past, but this time, we may not be able to. I just don't see you being able to head from the hospital to your apartment safely.

"Douglas and his brothers are already on me about that. They want me to move in with Douglas and his family so they can attend to me easier. There's talk of giving up my apartment," she said, wrinkling her nose as if she just smelled something noxious.

"Well, we can cross that bridge when we come to it. For now, let's sit in a chair and contemplate a brief rehab stay as a bridge to home—any home."

"That's fair. Okay, get out of here so I can rest up for my day of chair sitting."

"Good. See you tomorrow. Anything you need before I go?"

"No. I'm fine really. I'm perfectly fine." She shooed me away with her bony, knobbed fingers.

A few days later, Marion waved a pageant wave to me as I sat behind the desk at the rehabilitation center. She floated by like a guest of honor at a fourth of July day parade while grilling the EMS worker about his intentions with his girlfriend. "Was he going to propose or not? Women want a commitment . . . " she could be heard saying as they rounded the corner to her room. I smiled to myself as I finished charting my notes because from the sound of things, the old Marion was emerging with the same grace and resilience I had marveled at before. I sat at the desk a minute, giving the EMS workers time to settle Marion into her room. A crescendo of laughter reached the desk, which seemed to originate from an entourage of family members standing outside room 119. I strained to listen. The cacophony of sounds was confusing because it was out of place. Folks usually used their "inside voices" in these rehabilitation centers hyperconscious about disturbing other families. Was I hearing choking sobs or boisterous laughs? Were they arguing or kidding around? The sound seemed amplified given the recent renovation now that all the carpeting had been replaced by mahogany flooring.

"They're crying," clarified the unit clerk.

"They are?" I asked wide-eyed.

"Shouldn't someone help them? Shuttle them into the family conference room or something?"

"Doc, this isn't new. It happens every day around this time. It's gotten so that we don't even hear it no more."

"What's going on?"

"He's ninety-seven. On hospice. Kidney failure, I think," she said, not looking up from her chart dismantling.

"Ninety-seven?"

"Oh, Doc, please. This scene happens *every* day. You've never seen more family members in your life. The other day, the supervisor said they may be sister wives. You know, like polygamists—maybe he had twenty-four wives, fifty-four kids, one hundred twenty-five grandkids . . . you get what I mean."

"You guys are crazy. I'm glad I'm only around you two days a week."

"For real now. It's like the fun house at a carnival around here. Just when you think there's no more left, three more come outta the room."

"Did you say he was ninety-seven years old?"

"Oh, Lord Jesus don't get me started. The man's on hospice.

Didn't nobody tell these people that that means end of life, keepum comfortable, there's no turning back? I don't know how that poor man can get any peace the way they keep carrying on. It scares the other residents too. Admissions must have moved three residents already. Nobody wants a room down that hallway."

"I can imagine. What the . . . " I jumped startled by a loud popping noise.

"They're banging the wall. That's somebody's fist on the damn wall. I'll call maintenance. I'm not going down there. Jimmy will ask them to be quiet," she said. Jimmy was a menacing figure likening himself to Michael Clarke Duncan in *The Green Mile*. If Jimmy asked me to keep it down, you better know I'd be quiet in a hurry.

She reached for the phone,

"Hi, operator. I need Jimmy in maintenance . . . " That was my cue to grab my things and check on Marion.

"Hi, Miss Marion. How are you?"

"Oh, hi darling. I'm settling in, I suppose. I don't want to get too comfortable, you know. I mustn't overstay my welcome here."

"Nope. It's not a prison. We will spring you as soon as you regain your strength." After a brief exam and a rundown of her medications, I left her to a ringing cell phone.

"Douglas? Yes, I'm here. No. No need for you and Marcia to rush over. I'm perfectly fine. They'll be serving dinner soon anyway, so enjoy your evening and we can speak tomorrow. Yes, I have my cell phone charger. I think this thing has three bars. Oh no, that might be the volume indicator. Well in any case, I'm perfectly fine. Thanks for calling dear. You know where to find me. I can't go far." And she hung up. I'm glad I lingered outside the room long enough to hear her sound reasonably content.

On my way out, I thought I'd check on the Santa son and his father. It was approaching dinnertime so I could assess the "straw situation" as well. The room was dark and a straw poked up from the thickened apple juice container as the tray remained untouched at the bedside. I peered around looking for the Santa son. I'd thought he'd be here setting up the dinner tray. The father slept, contracted in bed, disinterested in eating.

I tapped him on the arm and said, "I'll get someone to help you with your dinner, ok?"

"Ok," he responded without opening his eyes. What did this fragile birdman dream? Perhaps he dreamt of a stronger, self-reliant time when he ate what he wanted when he wanted without the aid of a blender or a straw? I looked around the dark room. I wanted to see pictures of him in his youth or maybe a photo of his young family arm in arm at his son's high school graduation. Instead, a visual sweep of the room yielded end-tables baron of knick-knacks and a small closet with plastic hangers waiting for clothes.

"Hey Joyce," I said, seeing a personal care aide pass by the room on her way to assist another patient. "Can you help this gentleman with dinner when you're done with what you're doing?"

"Yes, Doc. No problem. I'll heat it up for him first 'cause I'll be in room 125 for a while. I'll get to him next though, I promise."

"Thanks Joyce. I appreciate it."

Weeks passed. Marion was still at the rehab center, as her convalescence wasn't progressing quite as she'd planned. Although still resilient of spirit, her body was weak, cachectic, and defeated. Douglas had begun the process of packing up her apartment with her reluctant permission. Just as Marion was preparing for plan B, the "polygamist" in room 119 was actively dying, and the birdman was ready to return home.

I sat at the desk next to the clerk and reached for the phone.

"The social worker asked me to call this fellow's son," I said out loud to no one in particular.

The unit clerk answered,

"Yep. I heard he'll be going home this week. She's trying to get him a hospital bed delivered."

"Maybe soon he can ride with his son with the wind in his hair or with the wind in his 'no hair'—whatever the case may be."

"You're bad, Doc," and she shook her head in exasperation. "That son hasn't been around lately." Before I could respond, he picked up the phone.

I decided to call the Santa son myself. "Good morning. This is Elaine Holt, the doctor from the rehabilitation center."

"Is everything alright?" he asked urgently.

"Oh, I'm sorry. Everything is fine. I'm just calling to tell you that your father's medical condition has remained stable and he's plateaued in physical therapy." Silence. I interjected with a rephrasing. "In other words, your dad is fine and he's made as much progress in therapy as he's going to make."

"Ok. That sounds good."

"Yes, it is. So, he'll be ready to go home on Friday. You'll be able to pick him up."

"Um. No, thanks," he said.

"What?" I asked.

"Huh?" he answered.

"I'm afraid I didn't understand you. I said that your dad is doing well and is being discharged on Friday and you'll be able to pick him up."

"And I said, no."

Confused, I asked, "Would you rather we arrange transportation for your father to get him to your home?"

"No." Now it was my silence that needed filling. He clarified, "No, I'm not picking him up, and no I don't need no transportation for him. I'm not taking him back. He's yours now." That was it. The doting Santa son was donating his father to us.

"You can't make this stuff up," I said out loud and relayed

the exchange to the unit clerk.

She deftly grabbed the phone receiver muttering, "I knew there was something off about them . . . Operator. I need the social work office." Her voice trailed off as she related the story and outlined the "obstacle" to the discharge plan. I sat, silenced by the recent news when Marion's nurse approached me and said that she was complaining of abdominal pain.

I waited a minute before heading to Marion's room collecting my thoughts. In the past, complaints of abdominal pain landed us in the hospital. I could arrange a "direct admission," sparing her the chaos of emergency room triage or we could wait things out here for a while if her condition wasn't too far along.

As I contemplated, the hospice nurse whizzed past the desk on her way to room 119. That gentleman's illness was coming to a close, and she'd been summoned by the rehab staff nurses to try to contain his family members. Like a hornet's nest just poked, a frantic, unsettled frenzy spilled out of his room into the hallway. A tall, strapping nurse herded a loudly sobbing woman in the crook of her armpit out of the room into the lobby while she whispered consoling platitudes. I suppose that the lobby, percolating with its large fish tank wall inset, was going to be the repository of these inconsolable relatives who at the same time required both comfort and segregation from other visitors.

Entering Marion's room, I said, "Oh, Miss Marion, are you causing trouble again?" somewhat exasperated myself at this replay of events.

"Certainly not on purpose, dear. Will you look at this belly of mine?" She tapped it in disgust.

"When are you due?" I asked snidely.

"Any minute by the looks of this. I'm virtually ten months pregnant!"

Frowning, I asked, "When did things get like this? I was just here a few days ago."

"I felt some twinges last night—no real pain, just twinges of discomfort, I tell you. It was nothing worth mentioning and now I'm like this." She burped, quickly covering her mouth. "And now the sounds that come out of me!" She shook her head. "Worse than a drunken sailor."

"Are you nauseated?" I asked.

"Just a little. Not as bad as it's been in the past, but I'm afraid it's coming." Placing my stethoscope on Marion's protuberant abdomen, I listened. I moved it around every few seconds in search of sound.

I heard the rustle of her fingers over her bed sheet. I heard the distant, persistent sound of an unattended call bell and the creek of a nurse's medicine cart making its way down the hallway, but I heard nothing from Marion's belly. Unhooking the earpieces of the stethoscope, I declared the verdict.

"I wish I could say that there was a heartbeat. Ha-ha." She forced a smile and waited. "For that matter, I wish I could say I heard bowel sounds, but I didn't."

"*Et tu Brute*," she said to her distended belly accusingly.

"What do you think, my friend? Is it time to go back?" I asked.

"Back where?" she asked.

"Back to the hospital."

"I'm not going back. I told you that last time," she said, all the while holding my hand. Despite her clarity, I felt the need to paraphrase the scenario to ensure our mutual understanding.

"Marion, I think that your bowel is obstructed again."

"I know."

"An operation may be necessary to open it up again."

"I won't do it."

"I know that you said that before, but sometimes people change their minds."

"Not me."

"Have you told Douglas?"

"I will. He knows that I have my mind made up. Dear, I'm tired. My body is tired." Looking out the window, but continuing to hold my hand, she said, "My life has been dismantled, but I find myself still here."

"So Marion, you understand that this will be our last illness together if you choose not to go back to the hospital?"

"I do." She freed her hand of mine so she could reach for her cell phone. "I need to call Douglas. You'll keep me comfortable, right dear? I don't want to suffer much."

"I will." I stood at her bedside waiting.

"It's ok, dear. Go ahead now and take care of sick people," she said, giving me permission to leave with her ringing cell phone at her ear. I blew her a kiss goodbye. As she did in return and she waved a pageant wave and said, "Douglas? Yes it's Mom. No, things are not fine, but everything is alright. I've made a decision, and I'll need to talk to you and your brothers . . . "

I walked briskly to catch up with the haggard hospice nurse who was just getting her things together to leave. She was probably questioning her choice of career after spending nearly the whole afternoon attending to the vociferous needs of the fish tank family. Touching her shoulder, I whispered, "You probably want to use that symptom-relief kit on yourself right about now?"

"I know. That was a challenge. Would you believe that they hadn't even had a funeral home picked out? The man was ninety-seven years old on hospice care. You'd think that one of those forty people were close enough to him to know what funeral home he wanted to use? I hope that he was peaceful. I feel like I spent more time in the lobby than at the bedside."

"I know. Let me thank you on behalf of everybody here. We really needed your help to contain the scene."

"Thanks. I'm glad it all worked out."

"Before you leave, I have a very special lady to tell you about. This case is much different." And she put down her bag, got out her pen and paper and with her coat still on, said, "Go ahead."

Marion asked the aide to help her dress and change out of the regulation Johnny coat.

"I can't have company wearing this thing," she could be heard saying. It wasn't long before the three brothers and their families assembled as Marion held court in her room. Towards the end of the evening, the daughters-in-law and grandchildren carpooled home, leaving behind Marion's three sons. So tall and broad surrounding her bed, they inadvertently shielded the view of her from hallway passersby. If you peeked in the room, just to make sure they didn't need anything, all you saw were the tufts of her mahogany hair puffing out above the overstuffed pillow. I don't know what they talked about, the brothers and Marion, but they did. They talked. They laughed a little. And then they each kissed their mother in turn. She gave them permission to leave and she gave herself permission to be alone. An unrepaired small bowel obstruction doesn't usually prove so swiftly fatal, but if Marion deemed it so, it was so. Marion was gone by the morning.

***

In my line of work, I always have a collection of sympathy cards on hand. I write them promptly to the surviving loved ones, often before there's any newspaper obituary announcement of the passing. After all, I'm usually in the know about the series of events, so there's no sense in delaying for formalities. I'm always surprised at how many sympathy gratitude cards I receive in return. I'm still holding out for some thank you notes for birthday and wedding gifts sent, but the families of those bereaved somehow find the strength to acknowledge my extension of sympathy. Maybe that's what the departed would have wanted.

Like weddings, funerals spotlight family pathology. I've been told that there's a wake crasher in every family. The aunt, cousin, or uncle who no one ever hears from, but who somehow appears in the regulation black dress or all-purpose funeral-wedding suit in a show of pious grief. I've often told my own mother that I want no such wake crashers at any event being held on my behalf. But as the circle of life would have it, my mother may predecease me and she therefore may not be the best custodian of this information (sorry, mother). So, I thank you in advance for allowing me the opportunity now to share some of my wishes.

A wake or a memorial often seems more about the living than about the departed. So often, these events degenerate into coffee-clutch gatherings where long lost relatives and friends catch up on mutual news as a casket flanks the head of the room. I don't think I like that concept. If some event is going to be held in my honor, I am inherently uncomfortable with not having a say in how it turns out. So, in other words, the best time to look for a job is when you have a job, and the best time to plan your funeral is when it's not imminent. I want no wake, no memorial, no funeral. I want my name, date of birth and date of death printed on a postcard with the following quotation beneath it:

Remember me with smiles and laughter,
Because that's how I'll remember you all.
If you can only remember me with tears,
Then don't remember me at all.

(P255 Confessions of a Prairie Bitch
—Alison Arngrim)

This was a poem read by actress, Patricia Neal, as she guest-starred on an episode of *Little House on the Prairie* written by Michael Landon. I want it sent via snail mail to everyone who may have come to a wake or a service and via email to those wake crashers who would have come out of obligation. This way, the mourners can hold a postcard in their hand for just a second and think of me and the others can either save it or delete it without the formality of donning funeral fare.

I came up with that idea shortly after watching the scene at the rehabilitation center. For me, the fish tank family of room 119 with their cringe-worthy cries and attention-seeking sobs became a caricature of grief. It was all very sad to behold. In essence, the staff and I watched the man in room 119 die alone in the presence of many. I wouldn't wish that on anyone. How did Marion do it? So many patients are on the carousel of illness, near recovery, illness, near recovery, but few are brave enough to stop the ride. How did she create a family of mourners—quiet, sincere, and graceful in their grief? I could never presume to know or even begin to generate an idea of how she did it, but I'm grateful that I was a voyeur into her peaceful passing.

And you may be wondering about the birdman? Well, he remained a member of the healthcare flock and there never was another Santa son sighting. I wonder who the staff will call when it is his time. Who "takes care of arrangements" when you've been abandoned by all who were supposed to have loved and cared for you? I believe that the birdman's passing will be quiet, but I don't know that it could be peaceful.

Chapter Eight

THE POWER OF THE "WORD"

Have you ever written something down
That later you'd regret?
Wishing that the reader
The meaning would forget?

Have you ever said out loud
Made an indiscretion with your words
Flinching at the memory
Hoping no one overheard?

Language is a tool
Used wisely, it's an asset
Its power lies in all of us
Far-reaching in its facet.

You can't escape the power
But denial you can try
"Words hurt" your mother used to say
That truth you can't deny.

A comedian who's on a rant
Toxic, racial slurs he's slinging
It's televised, memorialized
Then, the blues he will be singing.

A politician—future bright
To great heights this man might soar
One email, letter, essay scribed
A career in service—there's no more.

In the Age of Internet
A posting or a tweet
Can trail you for a lifetime
Unforgiving punishment you'll meet.

So what then is our recourse
If against "the word" you cannot win?
It must become your ally
Aware of meaning, watch its spin.

So perhaps reflect a moment
Before that YouTube speech you post
Reread the email that you wrote in rage
Press "send"—revenge then you will boast.

I was at a fifth grade graduation
They called it a "promotion"
The principal got up to speak
A silent crowd—there was no motion.

We expected he'd be boastful
Of the successes of the school
Accolades, accomplishments

Glowing test scores as a rule.
Instead the take home message
Was directed to the kids
About their life transition
Of grammar school they'd soon be rid.

As you enter middle school
As you grow and learn together
"Be kind to one another."
The memories of this time will last forever.

And that takes us full circle
A belief that we should hold.
To know the power of the words we use
Important for both young and old.

***

The ends of his button-down shirt flapped three-quarters of the way down his arms. He used his elbow stumps to shimmy himself onto the patient chair. The way his legs jetted out horizontally from the seat made me think at first that he was a little person, but his head and torso seemed appropriately proportioned. After a puzzling moment, I reconciled that he wasn't a little person. I went to shake his hand and awkwardly caught hold of the cuff of his shirtsleeve and the end of a stubby limb.

"I'm Steve," he said.

"Elaine Holt. Nice to meet you," I answered, assuming my position on the rolling stool and recovering from our awkward introduction. "Steve, what brings you?"

"Literally, a local cab service. Figuratively, my need for preoperative clearance."

"Fair enough. Let me start with a few questions, and we'll take a look at your pre-op paperwork afterwards."

"Sounds fine."

I knew that some of my questions would likely get answered if we ran through my standard history and physical exam inquiries.

"Steve, how old are you?"

"Sixty-three years young."

"And do you take any prescription medication?"

"I do. I have a list."

I wasn't sure how he was going to produce said list, but before I could offer my services to retrieve it, he craned his neck forward and pulled it out of his breast pocket with his pursed lips. The folded paper jetted out from his sealed mouth like a duckbill and with the end of his right arm, he clamped the paper and extended it to me. I rolled close to get it from him as the exercise of shimmying off the chair, waddling over to me, handing me the paper, waddling back over to the chair, and shimmying up, was too exhausting a production to even speculate about. *How did he do that?* I wondered to myself. His floppy, too long shirtsleeve still covered the ends of his arms, which I'd assumed were the stumps of amputation. But he seemed to pinch the paper's edge, almost like a claw? Well, I'd have to be patient . . .

"Thanks," I said, unfolding the list to have a look. Typed below were the medication names, routes of administration, frequency of use, once daily, twice daily, once a week . . . all meticulously noted. I remarked to myself: *No diabetes meds? No blood thinners?* One of the most common causes of amputations is peripheral vascular disease resulting as a complication from diabetes, smoking, or both and I didn't see any of the medications commonly used to treat PVD or its causes.

"I see the Methotrexate, folic acid, and a host of creams here?"

"Yes, that's for my rheumatologic condition and dermatologic condition respectively. Well, they're really one in the same."

"And what's that?"

"Psoriasis and psoriatic arthritis."

"Hmm," was all I could muster. *This degree of disability wouldn't have come from psoriatic arthritic, could it?* I asked myself. I thought I'd recently seen a television commercial with a professional athlete as spokesman for a new, injectable drug to combat the aches and pains of psoriatic arthritis, which restored him to his pre-affliction game. And wasn't there an actress on a commercial who was embarrassed into seeking treatment for her red, flaky patches of psoriasis by a naive, question-asking niece? She appeared blemish-free in the next frame, smiling and more confident. Was it that kind of psoriasis? Holding the list, I asked, "And what is your industry? I usually see these kinds of lists from engineers or old-time school teachers?"

"Close," he laughed. "I'm a library researcher, or maybe they'd call me an Internet researcher now."

"I don't think I know what that is," I confessed.

"I've spent the last thirty years doing library research for a law firm. They give me a series of questions and I give them the answers. I find supporting data, prior cases on a similar subject matter, and so forth."

"Really, I've never heard of that line of work."

"We may be a dying breed now, but I've made a thirty-year career out of doing what I'm used to doing: reading in a library."

"Fair enough." After going through the perfunctory social questions—never married, no kids, yes a smoker, half a pack per day, a social drinker only—we came to the reason for the visit.

"So you said that you're here for preoperative medical clearance?" I asked.

"Yes. I need the paperwork filled out before my surgery. The paperwork is under the medication list."

"What kind of surgery will you be having?" I asked, flipping the medication list over to view the preop form.

"I need a skin biopsy and likely removal of the lesion on my leg."

I glanced at his shortened pant leg and he must have anticipated my question because he volunteered, "I wear compression stockings, and I practically need a crane to get them on, so I'm going to need some help if you want to see."

Reaching for my gloves, I said, "I can help you out. I'd like to see the skin lesion, if I could." As I rolled his pant leg up to reveal a normal appearing knee, he elaborated on the treatment plan.

"We are doing the procedure in the operating room because the surgeon's not sure of its depth."

"Reasonable," I acknowledge. "Now may I just pull this black sock down?" He wasn't kidding that they were tight as the pattern of the stocking remained on his skin as I rolled the top of the knee high down. Copious flakes of skin fell onto the chair and the exam room floor and others were adherent to the inside of the nylon stocking.

"Jeez. I'm sorry about that. It's like winter in September in here."

"At least we don't have to salt, huh?" I replied unraveling his stocking to reveal a four-by-four bandage with paper tape applied to his sloughing skin.

"This is like one of those Matryoshka dolls. You know the Russian doll, within a doll, within a doll?"

"I do know what you're talking about. The suspense builds as you get to the littlest doll inside. Drum roll please . . . "

"I'm afraid to remove the tape. It looks like I could take a chunk of skin off."

"It looks like plenty of skin is already lying on your floor, so go for it."

Behind the gauze was a cauliflower-like lesion with dried blood at its center. "Nice," I noted.

"I thought you'd like that," he affirmed. "Do you want me to try to tape it up?"

"How would you do that?" I asked. "I wasn't sure if you had

hands underneath those sleeves."

"I do sort of." He invited me to raise his sleeve to reveal a claw-like remainder of a hand. There was the blunted vestige of an opposable thumb and shortened fingers that had webbed to work in unison.

"I don't think I understand. Now were you born with this deformity?"

"This?" he asked flapping his arm demonstratively from side to side. "No. I came into this world with hands, feet, legs and arms just like you or any other. This didn't happen until I was about twenty-four years old and it didn't stop until I was about thirty-five years old and like this."

"Oh, I'm sorry to hear that. I don't think I've seen anything quite like this before, so I thank you for indulging my questions." I had successfully reapplied a new four-by-four paper tape adhesive and was wrestling again with the black nylon sock.

"Questions are no problem for me. I told you. I've spent thirty years answering questions, so fire away."

"So you were born able-bodied with all of your limbs—hands, feet?"

"Yep."

"So what happened?"

"Well, no one really knows, but one thing I can tell you is I hurt. I always hurt, even as a kid. I never could play with boys in the neighborhood because my joints ached. I spent a lot of time watching stick ball games from my living room window. And that's when I discovered reading."

"To occupy your time indoors, you mean?"

"Well that and to get me outdoors."

"I'm not sure I understand."

"The boys in my neighborhood were always outside knocking a ball around or shooting a basket. I was never going to keep up with them, given my joint problems. I may have looked ok then, but I always knew something was wrong."

"It sounds a little isolating."

"A lot isolating, truth be told. I watched for a while, feeling left out. Then I started reading about the games: basketball, baseball . . . I became quite an aficionado. I started hanging around with some of the guys after school. They would be talking about a recent ball game, and I would chime in about the history of baseball and then I would throw in a fact or two about the rules. Pretty soon I was an authority on the games and when a question came up, they'd be like, "I don't know. Ask Steve . . . ""

"I'm glad you were able to integrate yourself like that. It's pretty impressive."

"Not really. You just have to know your audience. Most of them were a lot of fun—a great group of guys. Some of us are still friends today."

"Nothing like old friends, huh?" I affirmed.

"That's right."

Looking down at the pre-op paperwork, I noted that an EKG was required. "I see that we need to do an EKG. I'm not sure you can make the step up to the exam table."

Surveying the step from his chair, he concurred. "You'd have to hurl me up there. That could get ugly."

"Ok, well, let's not attempt it. We can try to perform the EKG with you seated." I left the exam room and the nurse completed the rest of the examination, including the phlebotomy and the seated EKG. He exited the office and chose to wait outside to grab a smoke before his friend arrived to pick him up.

"This might be a good time to quit," I shouted snidely as he exited.

"I don't have many vices left. I'm not giving this one up," he said, turning his back to the office, directing his attentions to the handrail and the concrete steps. Leading each step with his unaffected leg, he descended much like a toddler would.

One clunky, black shoe met the other on the step landing before he repositioned his arm further down the slanted railing and attempted the next step.

I wondered how he was going to light and hold a cigarette, but I imagined the trick might be similar to his medication list maneuver. I would process his preoperative paperwork and we would get together again at the hospital next week after the surgery.

One of the perks of outpatient medical practice is the parade of patients who come in and out each day sharing stories of personal trials and tribulations. Even if the patient is a reluctant communicator, a story can be gleaned from the looks and the laughs. A doctor, from his or her rolling stool, can enjoy the challenge of reading this spoken or unspoken narrative. Damian was another patient we saw later that afternoon. His story was difficult to learn, but worthwhile to know.

Damian was a high school art teacher with an unfortunate pear-shape who was coming in to discuss his weight-loss surgery. His love handles rippled over his synched belt and his thighs spread out on the seat to be pinched by the armrests. I imagined that plane travel could be a problem with his legs inevitably trespassing on the passenger's space beside him.

"Damian, how are things?"

"With me?"

"I don't see anyone else," and I mock-looked around.

"Oh, dandy. I saw the fat doctor shrink. She said that I'm competent to sign on for the surgery. And I saw the sleep guy who confirmed that I have sleep apnea and should be wearing that torture device apparatus at night."

"I hear from other folks that they feel more awake during the day when they wear the sleep apnea machine at night."

"Who wants to be more awake?" he said in response, posing the question just as much to himself as to me.

"Seriously, Damian. You have to fix what's in here," I tapped my head, "before the surgeons fix this," and I tapped my belly.

"I hear you, but I'm used to this," he said, tapping his own head.

"Just because you're used to it, doesn't mean it's healthy. Truly, I don't want you to go through with a potentially life-changing surgery only to eat through it. You could find yourself thirty pounds lighter in three months and ninety pounds heavier after a year. I don't want you to get discouraged."

"Too late, Doc. I'm there."

"Alright," I conceded, somewhat exasperated, "we'll come back to this topic."

"Promise?" he asked mockingly with an effortful smile.

"How's your mother?" I asked. She, too, was a patient of mine and had expressed concerns about her only son's upcoming surgery. Without revealing my own reservations, I promised her that I'd do my best to look after him.

"Ma? She's ok. Always doing something. There's a gaggle of kids around her at all times now that Janice and the rugrats are staying with her," he remarked, shaking his head. Damian was the first in his family to go to college and the pride and joy of his mother and sisters, who banded together in their matriarchal unit to raise the next generation of fatherless children.

"How's your class this year?"

"Oh not too bad. Art's required and not all the kids want to be there. They have to though."

"Is this year going better?"

"Than last year?!" he asked incredulously. "Any year could go better than last year."

The last academic year had been plagued by scandal, cruel jokes, and disciplinary action. Someone had hacked into the principal's personal email and had been sending Damian messages on her behalf. At first, they were congratulatory—

praising him on a job well done while sharing that he'd gotten rave student reviews about his art curriculum. He wasn't aware of any formal class rating system, but assumed it was one of many policies he was out of the loop on.

Later, the emails became more solicitous and suggested that they meet after school for coffee to "go over a few things." He wasn't much with words and fortunately, in this circumstance, answered in abbreviated forms like, "Thanks for the recognition," or, "I appreciate the compliment." He curtly agreed to meet at the local coffee shop at four p.m. He'd questioned it at the time, but quelled his concern with rationalizations about how he may be getting a promotion and how the discussion should happen off of school grounds. Arriving at the coffee shop, he'd bought two lattes and waited. It wasn't long before kids arrived, cell phones in hand. He looked away, sorry that this location had been suggested, unaware that it was such a popular after-school pit stop. He checked the time on his cell phone several times. 5:15 p.m. The lattes were cold and he felt foolish continuing to occupy a table for two. He emailed that he would be heading out and would be available in school tomorrow if a meeting was still needed. His answering machine was flashing by the time he got home. The high school psychologist had left a voicemail. She felt that it was important that Damian reach her as soon as he got the message. It was about the YouTube video.

Confused, he reached the psychologist who broke the news to him. The video featured Damian, voiceless, at the coffee shop with two untouched drinks. Sappy, sad music played in the background, and a young man's voice itemized all of the reasons a guy like Damian would get stood up: his size, his wardrobe, his distinctly undynamic personality, and so on . . .

Damian had come to see me shortly after the incident. The school nurse had sent him as she'd noted high blood pressure when she was evaluating him for a headache. He needed my permission before he could return to school. He was absolutely crestfallen and I had no words of consolation. The computer students who'd hacked into the emails were disciplined, as were those who filmed and posted the video. They were made to write an apology to Damian, which they handed to him in an envelope that he had yet to open. It was after that incident that Damian gained another fifty pounds and required long-term blood pressure medications.

"So when are you thinking about the surgery?" I asked.

"Maybe winter break. I've got sick days and, tacked onto a two week school hiatus, I should have some recovery time."

"You won't mind recovering over the holidays?" I asked.

"No. Holidays bum me out—my mom, my sisters, the kids all twittering around and then they fuss at me too. Asking if I want to join them going here or help them going there? It's another way of saying, 'get a life, you loser.'"

"Come on. You know that's not their intention. You are probably a *maaavelous* uncle," I said, drawing out marvelous like a Hollywood actress.

"Yep, one without a family of his own."

"In any case, I can see that you're working on your positive attitude."

He chuckled, flashing a super bright, white smile and remarked that he liked me because I gave him a hard time.

"Ok so what do I need to do for you next?" I continued.

"I think I'll need a medical clearance letter from you as we approach the surgery date, but not today. The sleep guy wanted you to check my blood pressure again 'cause he said it was high during the study."

"I can't imagine why when you have gooey stickers on your forehead and clinicians behind a mirrored panel wishing you into REM sleep. Sounds restful to me . . . " And I trailed off as I changed to a thigh cuff on our machine, preparing to recheck his blood pressure.

"It's hard as hell to fall asleep knowing that people are watching you or at least watching machines recording you."

I didn't answer as I listened to the blood pressure letting the cuff deflate.

"140/88. Not too bad. I wonder if they checked it with a small cuff?"

"Come to think of it, it did feel a bit like a tourniquet when they started pumping it up."

"Ok, so the blood pressure's fine. We have room to come down a bit, but I don't think we need to adjust any medications at this time."

"That's good. I wouldn't want to take any more pills than I have to down to the Bahamas."

Perking up, I said, "I didn't know about any Bahamian trip?"

"Yah, maan. I'm going to be working on my tan," he said facetiously. "I'm getting away for a little while—just three nights, four days. It's a package I saw online and there's a tour group you can join if you want."

"That sounds great. I want to hear about it when you get back, maybe see a picture or two."

"Sure thing. I'm planning on taking some fish photos with an underwater camera if I can sink low enough. Fat floats, you know."

Ignoring his self-deprecating jab, I said that I would really like to see those photos when he came back. Damian had started painting animals with oils. He'd told me once that oil paints permitted him to never finish. He could paint over shapes, change shades, rearrange still-lifes because oil paints were forgiving and absorbed one layer on top of another, never forcing commitment.

"Ok, chief, do you need any prescription refills before your trip?"

"I'll have to check, but I think I'm ok. I'm not leaving for a couple of weeks, so I'll call back if I need anything."

"Great. Safe trip and we'll see you when you get back." He shuffled in the front pocket of his portfolio briefcase rummaging for his car keys and I exited the exam room happy that I'd see some cool fish photos soon.

The rest of the week passed uneventfully and we were upon Steve's operation day. We were expecting a twenty-three-hour stay and a speedy discharge home. One of his buddies was going to drop him off at the same day surgery unit of the hospital and swing by the next day to retrieve him. Some of the stickball crowd were a couple of years ahead of Steve in school and were now newly retired looking for errand-like tasks to fill their free time, so Steve had assured me that he'd be able to round someone up to drive him.

I was in the middle of office hours when a visit was interrupted by a knock on the exam room door. Calls from my children, calls from hospital nurses, and calls from physicians all warranted knocks on a closed exam room door. I excused myself to take a call from Steve's surgeon.

"Hello, my dear."

"Hi. How'd it go?" I asked.

"Well, good and bad. He's stable and he's in recovery, but it's a squamous cell cancer. I'll have to wait for the final pathology, but I suspect we'll have to go back in to get wider margins."

"Shoot. That's going to really lay him up. He's not too mobile to start with."

"Yeah. I'm afraid we'll have no choice. I'll know more tomorrow. I just wanted to let you know that he's finished and the floor nurses will call you for orders when he's out of recovery."

"Ok. Thanks for your help. We'll talk soon."

I headed back to the exam room thinking that I could run

over to see Steve during our lunch break. When I got there, he had a visitor. His hospital room door was a jar and I made a "clopping" noise with my tongue three times and rapped in the air with my knuckled fist. That got the attention of Steve and his friend whose long legs extended in front of him to cross at the ankles. Retracting them a bit, he got up to a half standing position to greet me with a handshake.

"Hey, doc, this is my friend, Ken. He was going to chauffeur me home, but got bamboozled into a visit instead."

"Hi, Ken. Nice to meet you."

"Likewise."

"So, I hear you're staying with us for a few days. Some IV antibiotics and maybe another small surgery?"

"I don't know how small it's going to be. I guess we have to wait for the pathology results. I hear they have fine dining here."

"Menus and everything," I confirmed.

"I can bring you something, Steve. If that's ok with you doc?" Ken offered.

"Fine with me. You have no dietary restrictions," I said, turning my attention to Steve who was looking small in his huge hospital bed. "Meals high in protein are recommended for wounds."

"I can go to the Steak-n-Shake if you want. I can actually get Jim to do it. He's not doing anything important with himself nowadays and if he buys for the two of us, maybe he'll be more squared up on the money he owes us."

"Now that you put it that way . . . " Steve contemplated. I chuckled to myself at the easy banter between these two—a comfort borne out of a long friendship.

"It's time for that weasel to pay up," Steve concluded. Ken rose, a lanky, slightly hunched man of over six feet tall.

"I'm gonna step out and call him. Vanilla?"

"Yeah, that's good. Thanks."

"Nice meeting you, doc," said Ken as he walked out of the hospital room scrolling through his cell phone contacts looking for deadbeat Jim. I waved politely and turned my attention toward Steve. Approaching the head of the bed, I remarked to myself how child-like he appeared swallowed up in his oversized mattress. He was in a special bed that rippled in sand-filled waves to prevent skin breakdown. A trapeze hung from the ceiling to what should have been arm's length for the purposes of helping the patient pull himself up. No matter how many times Steve swatted his arms above his head, there was no way he was reaching that trapeze and likely couldn't have gripped it even if he were lucky enough to grab hold of it. It hung as an awkward, triangular reminder of his helplessness.

"This is quite a beach vacation here," I said, gesturing to the bed.

"Oh you mean this little shop of horrors they've got me in and the fact that it's hot as hell in here?"

"Yes. That's what I was referring to. Are you doing ok?"

"Yeah, I'm alright."

"Do you need anything? Is your pain adequately controlled?"

"I really don't have any more than usual. It's a little rough when they change the bandage on my leg, but I think that's only ordered for three times a day, so I'm fine. Everyone's been really good to me." Ken returned from his call and I used that as my cue to exit. On my way out, I heard Ken say,

"That cheapskate will be here around six o'clock. I told him I'd be back then, too, and not to take off with any part of my meal . . . " Muffled laughter followed me as I headed to the nurse's station to write in the chart. Steve remained hospitalized for a few days, receiving IV antibiotics and wound care until the final pathology report was in:

squamous cell cancer, invasive
extending to and including the margins of the specimen

I didn't evaluate a lot of pathology results, but you don't have to be a doctor to get the gist of "cancer," "invasive," and "including the margins." My next visit with Steve followed the surgeon's where he outlined the next surgery: the wide excision and debridement and the possible muscle flap closure. I found Steve halfway down into the center of the bed with his legs elevated higher than his chest.

Tilting my head almost ninety degrees to be at eye-level with him, I asked,

"How are you holding up? I heard that I just missed the surgeon's visit?"

"Well, I'm anything but up. I really need a boost. I'm afraid that I'm going to suffocate myself if I turn my head wrong and one of these sand dunes gets me."

"I'll grab a nurse and see if I can help you get upright," I said, about to exit.

"No, do it on your way out. They've been propping me up ever since I got here. I don't want to be a nuisance to them. So you talked to the surgeon?" he asked.

"I did. I told him that you're medically stable to go forward with another procedure if it's necessary, and it sounds like it is."

"Yeah. That's my understanding too. I think they're shooting for the day after tomorrow, but they're waiting for the OR schedule to be finalized." Looking around, I noticed that he had his laptop, a number of folders, and the latest fiction novel by a well-known author occupying his food tray.

"Are you planning to stay awhile?"

"Hell no. I want out of here as soon as possible despite the nice accommodations. I told the attorneys I work with that they're operating on my leg, not my brain. I can keep up my research unless I'm doped up from anesthesia, but that stuff doesn't stick with you too long."

"I'm glad you feel well enough to keep working."

"Listen, I have to. This surgeon's got me on bed rest, so if you don't have something else to occupy your mind, you'd go crazy. I don't need my leg to read."

"But you *do* need to be able to sit up. Unless you want anything else, I'm going to get you that boost."

"Sounds good. The nurses know where to find me."

"Good luck with the procedure."

"Yep. Thanks a lot."

Steve's surgery was successful by most accounts, but he was left with a gaping leg wound, which required elevation and immobilization. Steve was adamant about going home. He limped laboriously with two disfigured legs with foot stumps *before* the surgery, so the thought of him managing while non-weight bearing on one leg was discouraging. He said that he had his work at home and his resources there and that he'd made it this far without being institutionalized and wasn't going to settle for that now. When asked how he was going to manage his four-story walk-up, he briskly terminated the discussion by saying, "I'll figure it out." Herculean efforts by case management workers and physical therapists paved the way for his home discharge and off he went. He'd have regular appointments with the surgeon as an outpatient to follow the wound and I would likely hear from my colleague about how Steve's condition was progressing.

Weeks passed, and in medicine no news is good news. Things were quiet until I got an after-hours call from Damian's mother on a Friday night.

"Doctor?"

"Yes."

"This is Joyce, Damian's mother. I'm taking Damian to the ER." Her voice sounded tremulous and distant with a barely perceptible echo.

"Are you in the car?" I asked.

"Yes. I just picked him up from the airport. He came back

from that vacation of his and said he wasn't feeling well. He cut himself on a coral reef, and he was trying to keep it clean."

"Where did he cut himself?"

"In the Bahamas."

"No. I mean where on the body?"

"He said it was on his lower belly. Where it made it hard for him to watch it and care for it."

"Right. I understand. So you're going to the emergency room now?"

"I'm driving there right now. I'm about thirty minutes away. He's burning up and his eyes roll back in his head when he's resting. I keep nudging him awake just to make sure he can answer me."

"Ok Joyce. I'll call over there and tell them you're coming. Thanks for the heads up."

"Doc, I'm worried. He really doesn't look good and he's burning up."

"You're doing the right thing, Joyce. Just drive safely and get him to the emergency room."

"I'll try." She hung up.

By the time Damian got to the ER, he was in real trouble. His temperature was 104.0 with chills and low blood pressure at 74/palpable. He'd probably dutifully kept taking his blood pressure medicine while the infection was brewing. His pulse was fast—in the 130s—and he was growing listless. He had his age behind him as young men recover from septic shock better than their older counterparts, but things were still critical. By the time I arrived, his sisters had been contacted and were outside of his room comforting his mother. The critical care physician and infectious disease doctors were already making arrangements for his ICU transfer. Fluids hung wide open with pressors running to raise his systolic blood pressure. He was only minimally responsive with an oxygen mask covering his nose and mouth. I reached for the hand that didn't have the IV and he weakly returned my squeeze.

"Damian, it's me. Elaine Holt. You're in the hospital. You're in the right place. We are going to attend to your wound and treat the infection. You have to hang in there for me."

Groggy, he said, "Ok," and slurred, "Thanks for coming." I could tell that the history taking wasn't going to be informative from Damian and I'd have to turn to his mother for answers. A brief exam revealed an angry, reddened wound at the lower part of his abdomen approaching the groin with a purulent center and blackened edges. The nurse was covering it with a dry dressing and sealing it with adhesive tape. She had to lift his pannus with one hand and tape with the other. I offered to give her a hand, but by the time I'd gloved up, she was done.

"That took a little muscle," I commented.

"I know it," she said, "We're waiting for a bariatric bed and then he's set to go up to the ICU."

"I noticed that he barely flinched when you did that. What are you giving him for pain?" I asked.

"I didn't give him anything," she answered, gathering her supplies and leaving the ER exam room. I looked at the near lifeless Damian with his nonrebreather facemask, his cardiac monitor, and his IV lines and wondered how his mother was doing. I found Joyce pacing in a nearby hallway, no doubt distracted by her concerns. She startled when I came up behind her, but I didn't want to interrupt her silence.

"Joyce. How are you holding up?"

"Oh boy. Ok. This is not what I expected when I picked him up at the airport. He said he wasn't feeling well, but this caught up to him fast."

"Do you have any idea what happened?"

"I think I know some. About three days ago, when he was away, he said he cut himself on a coral reef. He didn't mention much about the cut. He was going on about how his waterproof shirt didn't come down all the way over his big belly and kept riding up. He was trying to get those underwater photos. I guess he cut himself where the shirt didn't protect him. That's really all I know. Then I picked him up from the airport like this," she said, welling up with tears. I heard the loud clicking of the wheels unlocking and two male transport aides deftly maneuvered Damian's big bed around the corner. They were headed to the ICU.

"Joyce, you follow behind them," I instructed. "You call me if you need to."

"You a relative?" one of the transporters asked.

"I'm his mother," Joyce answered and the transporter nodded that she should follow them.

When I went back to the office, there was a message from Steve's surgeon requesting that I call him back. Steve had missed two follow-up appointments.

"Hey, what's up?"

"Well, our friend, Steve, has been MIA."

"What do you mean?"

"He hasn't shown up for the last two follow-up appointments. I told him before he left the hospital that we'd have to watch that wound closely. It's deep and his skin integrity is poor. He's at high risk for complications."

"Steve's a smart guy. I'm sure he understood you."

"Of course he understood me. He just doesn't seem to be into it. He wants to do other things. He's in denial, Elaine. I just wanted to let you know where we're at. I had the ladies in my office reach out to him, and he said that he'd call back when he checked his schedule."

"What schedule? He works from home?"

"This is what I mean. The guy's in denial. I just thought I'd give you an update."

"Thanks. I really appreciate the call. I'm glad you filled me in."

"Ok. Let me know if he wants to get with the program."

"I will. Thanks again. We'll be in touch."

"Sure thing."

We'd probably be in touch sooner than he thought. When I was leaving the emergency room, the Infectious Disease consultants were conjecturing about necrotizing fasciitis and the possibility that Damian would need surgery. Maybe I'd be speaking to my surgeon colleague tomorrow about that.

I've only made three house calls in my career to date, but Steve lived in a studio in a collection of brownstone apartments not far from my office. My kids were on an overnight school field trip, freeing my evening of responsibilities. If Steve would have me, I'd pay him a visit. Remarkably, he was quite agreeable to my coming by, although he minimized any need to be checked on. He assured me that he was managing fine.

The entryway of the old building was narrow and dark. It may have made a good setting for those thirty-minute ghost story segments on TV. Mailboxes with untouched mail lined the foyer and I wasn't sure whether I should bring Steve's up to him. After some contemplation, I determined that it seemed too intimate a gesture, and I just started up the staircase empty handed. As I approached the fourth floor, I was distinctly aware of a putrid smell. I looked around for spoiled food or garbage, but the staircase was clean and well maintained. I'd imagined that tenants had already contacted the landlord speculating that a rodent had died in between the walls or in one of the vents. The saving grace was the weather. It had started to get cold and that may have tempered the odor a bit. I stood outside of Steve's apartment door and knocked.

"Come in. It's open," he shouted. The smell burned my nose as I entered, but Steve seemed unfazed. Maybe it was like carbon monoxide poisoning. Didn't they say that if you're in the room before the carbon monoxide leak, you can't smell the gas, but someone trying to save you would be aware of the fumes right away?

The stench of rotting flesh hung heavy in the air made worse by the sauna-like temperature in the apartment. Steve's steam heater cracked and whined, trying to reach its thermostat setting. I knew that cold temperatures exacerbated his arthritis, so it was no surprise that he kept the place hot. What was a surprise was the stink. I was certain it was his wound. He literally was decomposing, but seemed mercifully unaware. I spent a brief period of time trying to cajole him to the surgeon's office reminding him of the severity of his condition. He said that he'd think it over once he got to a breaking point in his project. I knew how far to push it and this was far enough. I turned my attention to his built-in book shelves and antique desk equipped with quill and ink.

"You don't actually write with that do you?"

"No, wise guy, I don't. I couldn't pick it up anyway. It's a period piece. It goes with the desk." As befitting a studio apartment, the bedroom, dining room, and TV room were all in one. A sliding board extended from his bed to a platform and at the end of the platform would sit his locked wheelchair when not in use.

"That's a nifty setup," I commented, gesturing to the sliding board.

"Courtesy of home physical therapy. I've been trying to keep my leg up, but truth be told, I couldn't walk on it if I tried. They've equipped me with this sliding board to make the bed to wheelchair transfer. I spend most of my time in the chair now."

"Steve, you don't have to tell me, but how did you get up here to this apartment? I'm sure the Fire Marshall would be thrilled. This is like the opposite of 'I've fallen and I can't get up.' 'I've gotten up and I can't get down.'"

"You ought to do stand up," he chortled. "You really want to know?"

"I do."

"Ken carried me. It was a King Kong and Ann moment. I told him I'd marry him if he got me over the threshold. He said he was already spoken for. He and Mary were married forty years last spring. I was one of his groomsmen."

"I'm sure you were very dapper."

"I was."

"Has Ken been over recently?" I couldn't imagine that Steve had had any visitors of late because it would be impossible to ignore the odor in the apartment. I don't have a good sense of smell, so I am told by my office nurse, and even I found it a little overwhelming.

"No. He's been wanting to come by, but I've told him that I'm backed up on some of my projects. We go to lunch with the guys on Fridays, but now that I'm in the chair, I feel a little funny about it. Ken's offered to get me in the truck and that way we could fold the chair in the back, but it seems like a lot of trouble to me. He calls, though, to check in. So do the other guys."

"That's nice. You have a fine group of friends."

"They're ok," he said with a smile of satisfaction.

"Will you please call me if you change your mind about the surgeon's follow-up? I'll help facilitate the appointment."

"I know you will." I took that non-answer as my cue to leave. "I'll just show myself out, Steve."

"Listen, thanks for coming by. It was really nice of you."

"No problem. Call me if you reconsider."

"Will do. Careful going down the stairs. They're tricky when it starts to get dark."

"Thanks," I said and waved goodbye. I scurried down the steps quite skillfully, motivated by my desire for some fresh air. For the sake of Steve's pride, I hoped that the landlord would take his time searching for that dead animal.

I visited Damian the next day in the ICU. He had done well overnight and was more alert the next day. I approached his bedside.

"Hey trouble-maker. How are you feeling?" He stared back at me, eyes wet and sullen like a basset hound's. "Listen, I'm not making light of anything. I'm just relieved to see you looking a bit better." Again, a wordless stare. "Damian, what's up?"

"They just told me I need surgery. The antibiotics stabilized me overnight, but the wound's getting bad fast." I came to learn that the critical care physician had reached out to my surgeon colleague and he was going to put Damian's case on as an add-on that same day. "They think I have necrotizing fash . . . something. It doesn't sound good."

"Well, it's not good, but it's manageable. You're young and your overnight response is a good omen. Things are probably going to get worse before they get better, but you have to be positive."

"You know what this means, don't you?"

"No. I don't know what you're talking about."

"My other surgery. The one over December break. That's not happening. I already asked. This wound has to heal first and I'm going to be left with a man-made shark bite out of this blubber belly. They said it could take nine months to heal that and then we can talk about the fat guy surgery."

"Damian, you almost died. You're still not out of the woods, but we have to take this one day at a time, one procedure at a time. Let's get through the surgery today, ok?" No answer. "Damian, has your mother been in yet today? She'll be thrilled to see you looking better."

"Visiting hours start at ten," he reported, his voice monotone as I glanced at the clock, which read 7:30 a.m.

"Well, I'm sure she's going to be happy." No smile. No response. "Damian, I'm going to leave you. Good luck later today.

You're in good hands, so please try to be positive. Your *outlook* can determine the_*outcome*. Remember that." No answer—just basset hound eyes. I left the ICU feeling more tired than when I'd arrived and I would wait to hear from the surgeon about how things went.

Damian made it through the surgery and was left with an abdominal wound the size of a baby's head. It was going to have to heal from the inside out and would require daily packing, wound vacuum applications, and a lot of care. He applied for short-term disability from work, and his wound needed extensive home and nursing care after what turned out to be a two-week hospital stay. I knew that I wouldn't see him in the office again for a while and upon his departure from the hospital said, "Damian. When you're up and moving around a bit, I want you to show me those fish photos."

"If there are any worth seeing," he added.

"I'm sure there are. I'd love to see what you're going to do with them. I'm not too artistic myself, so I really do want to see what you're going to create."

"Ok," he muttered to himself.

"Seriously. Don't blow me off. I really want to see what you shot so when you're back on your feet, try to remember to bring some to the office. Ok?"

"Ok," he said, a little louder this time. "Thanks for everything."

"No problem. Just keep getting better. One day at a time." And I left his exam room knowing that it would be months before I'd see him in the office again unless, of course, a complication arose. He'd be too busy with wound care and surgical appointments to come for routine visits and visiting nurse services were set to see him at home for blood pressure monitoring and the like so I'd probably get telephone progress reports from them.

On the way out of the hospital, my office texted me, "Ken called. Said Steven's not right." Something was lost in the text translation and I ducked into one of the nurse's stations to use a landline.

"Hi. It's me. What does that mean?"

"Ken said that he called Steve to say hi and he sounded all spaced out on the phone, said he was out of it."

"What did he do?"

"He told me he called 911 and was going to meet the EMS guys at his apartment. He wanted to let us know."

All I could imagine was the EMS worker breaking the door down sure from the smell that his patient was dead for days only to find Steve, sleepy, sitting up in his wheelchair. I stayed at the hospital, completing some medical records because Steve would likely be wheeled into the ER in under twenty minutes given his proximity to the hospital. It made sense for me just to wait. I'd make it a point to thank Ken for the heads up as it streamlined my morning plans.

Sure enough, within a half an hour Steve's name popped up on the computer screen noting his location as ER triage and the diagnosis: CHANGE IN MENTAL STATUS. I made my way downstairs to find Ken giving the receptionist Steve's identifying data: full name, birth date, address and so on. I waited for them to be finished before asking him what he knew.

"Hi, Ken. Thanks so much for contacting EMS. Did they have to break the door down?"

"Yep, they did. We knocked. I called for him, but he didn't answer. They broke the door down and found him in bed, kind of groggy. They were able to wake him up, but something's not right."

"Did they do anything once they were inside? Like give him medicines or anything?"

"No, all I saw the guys do was take his blood pressure and give him oxygen. They were worried he'd had a stroke or something and called over here. I think that's why they got him in so fast."

Steve wheeled by on his way to a CAT scan, no doubt under the direction of the neurology stroke team. He looked comfortable, like he was sleeping, but something was definitely wrong because the stretcher got jostled pretty ungracefully to make a tight corner to the radiology area and Steve didn't so much as flinch.

"And, Doc, the EMS guys wanted to know what the stench was. The apartment really had a funny smell. They weren't sure if that had something to do with Steve's condition. Like was he poisoned by fumes?"

I didn't have the heart to tell him that the smell was coming from Steve and that it wasn't related to his mental status change. Just then, the receptionist returned with an "intent to treat" form and directed her attention to Ken.

"Are you a family member?"

"No, a friend."

"Are you authorized to sign documents for the patient?"

I took a step back and distractedly checked my cell phone email while she completed her questions, but I was surprised to hear Ken say, "Yes." That seemed to perk up the receptionist's ears too.

"Yes? So, sir, you are authorized to sign this 'intent to treat' document on behalf of the patient?"

"I think so. I'm his POA."

"Ok, that's fine. So, sign here and here and please put your name and contact information in the box marked Power of Attorney."

I don't know why I was taken aback by that. I suppose all those years working in a law office had taught Steve a thing or two about crossing his "T's" and dotting his "I's." Steve's parents had predeceased him and he'd neither married nor had children so a good friend like Ken was a perfectly reasonable choice for an appointed decision-maker, but most people don't have the forethought or presence of mind to choose someone for this role.

After Ken had finished with the receptionist, he turned his attention back to me and said, "Maybe I should give you my cell number if you need anything. If Steve's going to be out of it for a while, you may need to end up calling me." I gladly took his number and offered him my business card in exchange as he, too, may have questions while the mystery of Steve's condition unfolded. Ken stood silently for a while, aware that he had just signed onto a great responsibility.

A battery of tests were performed and it became clear that Steve had not had a stroke. Blood tests revealed an abnormally high calcium level: thirteen and climbing. There aren't too many causes of hypercalcemia and in Steve's case, CAT scans revealed the worst possible one—metastatic cancer. The oncologist on the case took one look at Steve and explained that it was uncustomary to give chemotherapy to the bed bound. He could probably lower the calcium enough with some drug cocktail for Steve, to become a little more lucid, but those efforts weren't likely to change the outcome. He asked that I clarify the patient's wishes and let him know if he could be helpful. His parting words were, "You know, hypercalcemia's not the worst way to go."

I left the hospital grateful that I'd soon be seeing some office patients with appointments for physical exams, upper respiratory infections, and follow-ups. I'd call Ken in between visits and give him the bad news. Steve, the man who made a living by reading, who had integrated himself into an able-bodied world by talking, had just lost his ability to process words. I would defer to Ken about the oncologist's offer to chemically arouse Steve. We'd only do that if Ken felt there was something left unsaid. Otherwise, Steve would be allowed to fall deeper and deeper into a hypercalcemic sleep.

I was told by the nurses that night that a group of guys came to visit Steve and some of them brought their wives. They were quiet in the room, occasionally whispering to one another as though not to disturb him. Earlier in the day, the nurses had done a heroic job at sanitizing Steve's wound and the odor was replaced by wafts of Lysol and irrigation solution. Ken signed documents on Steve's behalf, placing him on comfort measures only. He required no morphine and no sedatives. His calcium-induced stupor made for a wordless fade-away.

The next couple of weeks were uneventful in the office. I'd bumped into Damian's surgeon on a number of different occasions and each time was met with a thumbs up and a debriefing of the wound care progress. Damian was being taught to change his own dressings although the location and extent of the wound made it difficult to be fully self-sufficient. Visiting nurses and home health aides were still coming by to assist him with his personal care needs. I knew from his time in the hospital how much he loathed the attention, despite the nurses' reassurances that they were there to care for him. I wondered whether he felt well enough to do any painting while he was home. That might help bring him out of his funk. On one of my last meetings, the surgeon did confirm my suspicion regarding the duration of the healing process. "Wounds don't tell time," he said.

It would likely be nine months before the area healed and that included a possible skin grafting procedure in between. This delay would devastate Damian, I thought to myself, and I pledged that I would reach out to him soon. I didn't have to wait to hear from him because Damian called the office looking for a refill on his Metoprolol, his blood pressure medication. I intercepted the receptionist and said that I'd pick up the call.

"Damian, we were just thinking of you. How are you doing?" I asked, envisioning those basset hound eyes.

"Not too bad," he answered—very un-Damian response. His voice sounded strong too.

"Really?" I asked, almost disbelieving. "How's it going?"

"Ok. The visiting nurses have all been nice. No complaints."

"Have you been able to do any painting? Have you done anything with those fish photos?"

"Some and no."

"What do you mean some?"

"I've picked up my oil paint brush here and there, but I'm not finished."

"It seems like the design is to never finish. Maybe you should just stop and start a new one. Share the old one."

"Maybe." A man of few words. I've always thought that a lot went on in his head, but the dialogue was conducted three-quarters of the way with himself and never made it to the listener.

"Well, think about it. What can we do for you?"

"I need a refill on my blood pressure medicines."

"Do you want them delivered or is someone going to pick them up?"

"My mother can probably pick them up. And, I have a new prescription plan. I can get a ninety day supply."

"No problem." I jotted the information down on one of our telephone sheets, saying out loud to myself, "Metoprolol Succinate ER 100mg daily. Ninety tabs, no refills."

"That should do it," he acknowledged.

"Ok, Damian. Keep getting better. You sound strong. I want you to call if you need anything."

"Yep."

"What's yep? Really. Call if you need anything since it could be a while 'til we see you again."

"Will do."

"Bye, Damian."

"Bye, Doc."

The ladies in the office asked in series how Damian was doing and each seemed genuinely happy to hear that things were looking up. That was a good way to end the week and in a few hours we'd be closed for the weekend.

Fridays and Mondays are often the two busiest days in the healthcare industry as folks want issues resolved before the weekend or hold out waiting until Monday to address them. This Monday was no exception. The nurse and I darted back and forth between exam rooms staggering EKGs and blood draws with doctor-patient visits. I was in an exam room with a patient when there was a knock on the door. I excused myself and the receptionist, appearing pale, said, "The police department is on the line. It's an officer about one of our patients. He said that he wasn't authorized to tell me who."

"Ok. Thanks."

I poked my head back in the exam room, laying out a changing gown and lap drape and instructed the patient to go ahead and get changed while I took a quick phone call.

"Hello."

"Is this Dr. Elaine Holt?" I could feel my heart beating faster. I'm the kind of person who gets nervous if I see a police car in my rear-view mirror, so speaking to the police automatically increased my anxiety level.

"Yes," was all I could muster.

"Doctor, I wanted to call and inform you about the death of one of your patients."

"Ok," I squeaked.

"We are at the home of Damien Brown and the paramedics have just pronounced him."

"What? Are you kidding?" I asked foolishly.

"I'm afraid not, ma'am."

"Do you know what happened? Are you allowed to tell me?"

"Yes ma'am. I'll tell you what I know. We were called to the scene by the victim's mother. She arrived at the door for a visit and when he didn't respond, she called the police."

"How did you know to call me?"

"Well, it seems as if the victim took his own life. A nearly empty pill bottle was found near his bed with your name on it. It says . . . Metopro . . . Well it says here generic for Toprol XL."

"Metoprolol Succinate ER," I clarified.

"Yes, that's it. He didn't leave a note, but this is being treated as an apparent suicide. I just wanted to inform you. You won't be called on to sign the death certificate because this is an M.E. case."

"Thank you so much for letting me know what happened," I said, my voice cracking.

"I'm sorry to have to give you bad news, doctor."

"I know. Thanks again." With my head in my hands, I thought of Damian's mother pacing outside his door waiting for the police to arrive, fearing that her son had been overcome again by infection. I'm sure that she, like so many others, never suspected that he would take his own life. He left with no note and no warning. I didn't know how many blood pressure pills would have amounted to a lethal dose, but certainly, the ninety that I'd called in would have sufficed.

Damian never felt that the power of the written or spoken word was his to access. Maybe that's why he never opened the letters of apology written by those trouble-making students. Reading their remorseful letters might have freed him of some anguish. Communicating with his colleagues might have earned him a friend or two—maybe even someone with whom to share his extraordinary artistic talent. Instead, I speculated that his photos and paintings would get boxed up and stored in a dark closet as the sight of them would be too much for his grieving mother. Just then, the nurse, unaware of the telephone conversation, came into my office and asked whether I was going back into the exam room or whether she should go in. I asked that she go in. This bought me a few more minutes to digest the news. Later, I would tell her the story of Damian's death.

***

I will never know why the Damians of the world wordlessly slip into isolation or why the Steves of the world integrate themselves in spite of great odds. But I'd like to know. Of course, mental health, circumstance, good fortune, and forces we don't understand can all contribute to a person's ability to cope, but language skills, both written and spoken seem to play at least some role in the process. If Steve wasn't so well read, could he have integrated himself among the neighborhood stickball crowd? Could he have earned a living and been self-sufficient despite his profound physical disability? And perhaps even more curious, could he have engendered the love and support of friends who were like family to him despite his limitations and illness? Would things have ended differently for Damian if he felt that he could access others through language? Both his and Steve's passings were wordless, but Damian's seems so unfinished. Of course that is the nature of an untimely and unnatural death, but so much was left unsaid. The torment of isolation is unlikely to be erased by accessing the written or spoken word, but I wonder if it can be eased? In Damian's case, as in so many others, we will never know, but I am left at least wondering about the power of language.

Most of us want our opinion heard, if not valued, and one way to affect that is by expressing it in print. Internet websites have become a popular forum for the otherwise voiceless to gain self-expression, but I caution that both children and adults reflect on the power of the written word before taking to the keyboard. A topic that can get a rise out of my physician colleagues is the "rate your physician" websites that have grown popular. Although most consumers understand that these forums for expression are completely unregulated and that anyone is free at any time to post anything, we still find it hard to read with skepticism because, in a reader's mind, the opinions are authenticated by the very fact that they are printed. I too fall victim to wanting to believe what I read.

So, perhaps we should be careful about what we write down not only because in the age of the Internet, words are indelible, but also because people have the natural instinct to believe what they read. There are countless actors, politicians, and businessmen who fall from grace because of a letter or an email transmission. In this regard, we, all of us, are writers and have a responsibility to value the power of words.

Epilogue

Doctors are like fruit. They can ripen over time, but they are susceptible to rot.

I remember a senior colleague of mine once saying, "Medicine is a high burn-out field. You have to pace yourself. "Looking back, he may have been responding to my almost manic New York City speed transplanted awkwardly into the smoother, slower rhythm of things in his office as I had just taken a private practice job down south. Cross-cultural differences in gait aside, I knew what he meant and have recited those words to myself more than once as a cautionary tale. Over the years, I've had the opportunity to speak with folks in service professions from law enforcement to teaching to medicine and many come precariously close to "soul decay" over time. They grow disenchanted with their work, jaded by the politics of their field, and mournful of the wide-eyed do-gooder they once were. Well, altruism alone does not a career make and you never want to be a casualty of your own enthusiasm.

These pearls of wisdom are well illustrated in interviews I've conducted with graduate students. I've had the occasion to hire graduate students in need of some work and desirous of some extra money as they pursue their respective degrees. The face-to-face encounter is the only way to weed through resumes that all seem to look alike with prominent GPA reportings and itinerizations of obligatory volunteer work. I hope that I've honed my skills as an interviewer, learning to stay silent during awkward pauses rather than self-indulgently injecting my nervous talk to fill them. I usually ask open-ended questions like, "Name an experience you're particularly proud of," or, "Now, name an experience that you're not particularly proud of." I usually wrap up with something generic like, "What makes you want to enter the medical field?" Nothing shuts down the exchange faster than a response like, "I chose a career in medicine because I really want to help people."

Oh pleaaase! Groans the thought bubble in my head. I hear *The Price is Right* music in the background, the three-note sound for the loser, the one who chose wrong and is about to be escorted off stage empty handed. Although a bit dramatic, I envision myself standing up from behind the desk, fists slamming down like gavels shouting, "That's not the truth. You can't handle the truth!" I'll argue that we've arrived at a "dialogue DNR"—Do Not Resuscitate. Most doctors go into the field because they want to help people. That sentiment is real, but it alone is not enough to ward off "rot."

Although physicians have the potential to rot over time, they have the potential to ripen as well. One of the great seducers of a career in medicine is the notion that doctors can get better with age. In my youth, I watched more than one fifty-something executive discarded in the prime of his/her career, a casualty of the ageist business community. In medicine, there's a sense that physicians improve with time, gaining at once clinical experience and humility. So, you're not put out to pasture because you're fifty-five years old with graying temples. That's a perk. Because physician schooling is so lengthy, you really don't set out on your first job experience until you are between thirty and thirty-seven years old, depending on the area of medical specialty. Taking this into consideration, it is essential that we value our senior colleagues. They've seen a lot, done a lot and learned a lot. I'm glad that wisdom and experience are still celebrated among physicians. I'd argue that other industries could take a page out of our book with respect to this. I've seen a lot of disease, devised a lot of treatment plans, and, most valuable, have had a lot of doctor-patient encounters. I have my career as a community physician to thank for those experiences.

I was recently asked back to my residency program to participate in a panel discussion on "life after residency." I was honored and delighted to be invited back to the "mother ship," but was frankly surprised that I was. I hadn't had any real professional contact with my residency program for almost two decades and surmised that the folks in charge must have gotten to "H" in the phone book and started firing off calls and letters. Once I arrived at the lecture hall, it became clear why I had been tracked down. The panel was made up of four guest physicians: an academic doctor, a hospitalist, a hospital-employed clinic doctor, and me. I joked to myself that they had to go back two decades and cross state lines to find a private practice doc to join the panel.

I enjoyed fielding curiosity questions from this bright and charitable audience and sharing my experiences in private practice with those impressionable, young doctors reaffirmed for me my happiness with my own career choice. I don't know that I was able to recruit any of them into private practice medicine, but I hope that I told a few good tales and that they enjoyed a few good laughs during the session. I cautioned the group to remember that you don't get lobotomized after you leave the ivory tower and that the everyday patient is capable of teaching you a thing or two.

Although I don't remember the exact wording of the question, one of the residents in the audience asked me why I went into medicine. This was a bit déjà vu as I've tortured many a graduate student interviewee with the same question. After I thought for a moment, I said, "Because I never tire of people and their stories."

At the end of the session, one of the other physician panelists said to me, "Well if medicine doesn't work out, you can always do this. You tell a good story." I was appreciative and graciously thanked him, but I knew that this wasn't entirely true. If I wasn't a physician, I couldn't tell a good story.

I remember being really excited leaving the panel discussion that day. If I had been entertaining or informative, I was glad, but I knew that I'd come away from the experience with more than any of the residents had likely gleaned. I realized why I had not fallen victim to "physician rot." I truly never tire of people and their stories. I am excited at the prospect of each patient encounter because I never know what I'm going to get. Sharing stories and fielding resident questions about my private practice career illuminated for me much of my motivation for staying in it. I enjoy the ride. I enjoy the triumphs, reflect on the losses, and love reminiscing enough to recount the tales.

I decided then that I would try to do my career in medicine justice and attempt a work of medical writing. I'd try to write a book that would be a giant thank you note for the amazing career I've had and hope to continue having—ripening over time.

ACKNOWLEDGMENTS

I'd like to thank John Koehler and the team at Koehler Books for taking the project on. It is always a leap of faith to invest in a new writer and I appreciate the show of support. I would also like to thank my editor, T Campbell, whose expertise and efforts have helped make this book better.

I would like to thank my dear friends and "readers," Marilyn Caccavella and Nelson Chen, along with my sister, Natalie Holt, for their input and support during the pre-publication process. A special thanks goes to Alexandra Alvarez for her computer savvy and her willingness to go on this wild ride with me. Along the same lines, I thank Ashley Bartscherer for lending this project the final enthusiastic push it needed.

I'd like to acknowledge in general, the physicians and teachers in medical schools and residency programs who dedicate their lives to shaping future doctors. Special gratitude goes to my parents, Carmela and Bill Holt, whose selfless dedication to the education of their children helped make this book possible. Thank you to my daughters, Alexandra and Isabelle. You are my inspiration.

And last but not least, I must thank my husband, John, whose endless support and encouragement propelled this project to completion. Thank you for believing in me, and I, for one, am grateful that this manuscript became a book because if it hadn't, I would have never heard the end of it. Thank you!